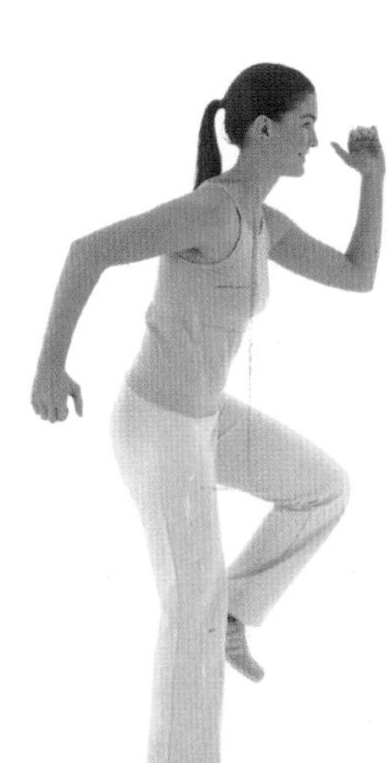

body sculpting

First Published in Great Britain in 2004 by
Hamlyn, a division of Octopus Publishing Group Ltd
2–4 Heron Quays, London E14 4JP

Distributed in the United States and Canada by
Sterling Publishing Co., Inc.
387 Park Avenue South, New York, NY 10016-8810

ISBN 0 600 60864 6

A CIP catalogue record for this book is available from the British Library

Printed and bound in China

10 9 8 7 6 5 4 3 2 1

Note

Whilst the advice and information in this book is believed to be accurate, neither the author nor the publisher will be responsible for any injury, losses, damages, actions, proceedings, claims, demands, expenses and costs (including legal costs or expenses) incurred or in any way arising out of following the exercises in this book.

hamlyn

body sculpting

Chrissie Gallagher-Mundy

contents

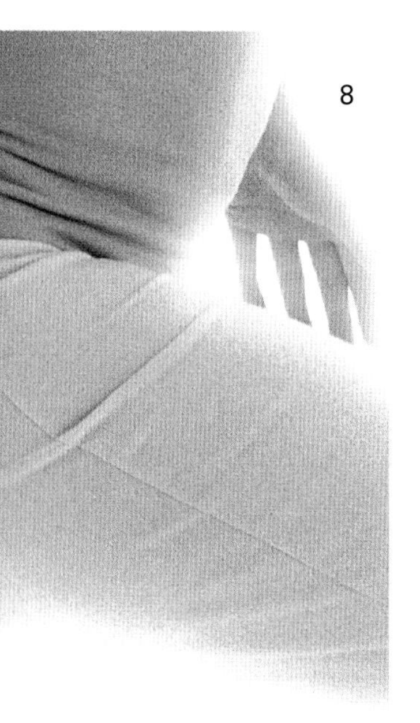

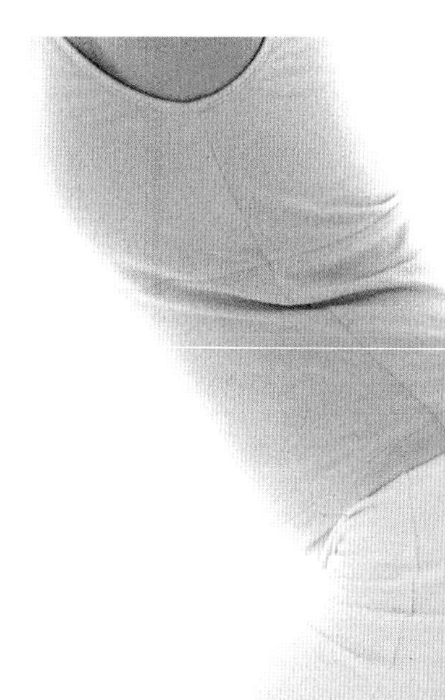

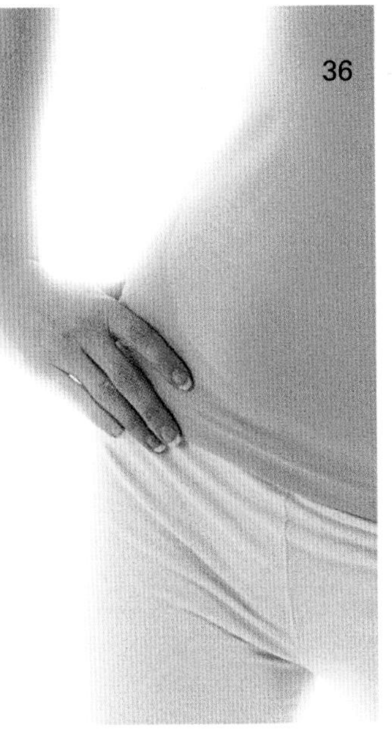

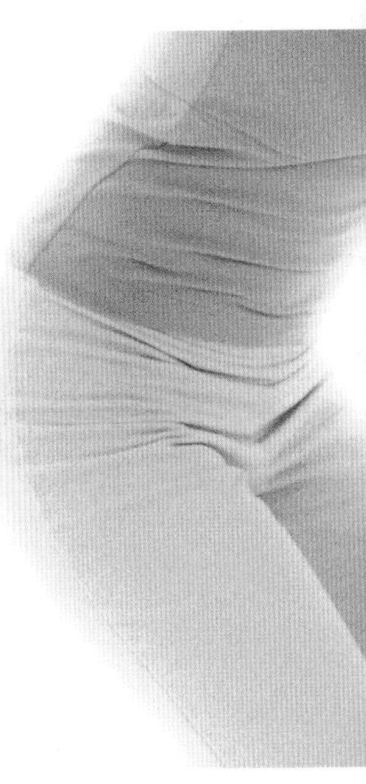

Introduction

Humans come in different shapes and sizes. Some societies favour men and women who look sleek and slim while others prefer more rounded figures. Many people are body conscious and the logical follow-on is to ensure that they look after their bodies and hone its natural shape towards their perceived ideal.

In the Western world food is plentiful. While it's easy for us to eat nutritious food, our busy modern lifestyles have led us to consume greater amounts of fast and ready-to-eat foods. Consequently, it's easier now than ever to take on board too many calories. And excess calories are stored as fat. Physical activity also becomes easier to avoid; with modern inventions such as the vacuum cleaner, the washing machine and the car, we can gain a few unwanted pounds almost without noticing. Bear in mind that it's the combination of healthy eating (which provides your energy) and regular exercise (which burns the energy) that will give you your best body shape.

On the plus side, however, our modern lifestyle also provides us with the means to take our bodies in hand and get them back into shape. Most people will have areas of their body they are happy with and areas they are not. Since few of us have unlimited time for endless amounts of exercise, when you do work out it needs to count. *Body Sculpting* is specifically aimed at helping you focus on the areas you need to improve. It will help you identify your particular problem areas and guide you towards the right muscle exercises to target and improve specific areas of your body.

The body-sculpting programme outlined in this book involves a two-pronged attack:

1

Firstly, you work on specific muscles to strengthen them. By working them hard you build your muscle mass, which means you burn more calories – even when you're not exercising.

2

Secondly, as you stretch and lengthen your muscles after each muscle-building, or toning, session you ensure that the main belly of the muscle is long and lean, rather than bulky, thereby enhancing the mobility of your whole body.

Improve your shape
The toning and stretching exercises throughout the book, combined with the cardiovascular (CV) exercises to help reduce your levels of body fat, will result in a difference to the way your body looks – your shape will become more balanced and honed.

The book contains workouts for four specific body areas that people often want to improve:

- Stomach and waist
- Bottom and hips
- Legs and thighs
- Arms and upper body

Six-week goal
There is a six-week programme devoted to each body area which, if followed regularly, can make a big difference to your shape.

Five elements
Each programme is split into five different areas of exercise, which should be performed in the following sequence;

1 Warm-up
to mobilize the joints and ready the body for exercise

2 Cardiovascular
to burn fat and improve the function of your heart and lungs

3 Balance
to improve posture and tone the core muscles

4 Toning
to improve muscle tone

5 Stretching
to enhance mobility

Notice the difference
Each programme is designed to build in intensity from week to week over the six-week period so that your muscles are constantly challenged as you become stronger and more shapely. You should perform the exercises three or four times each week to get the maximum benefit, and the routine should take you no longer than 45 minutes so that it fits easily into a busy lifestyle.

At the end of each six-week programme you will notice an increase in your strength and balance as you go about your daily life. You will be more alert in mind and body as your blood is pumped around the body more effectively and you will see an improvement in your appearance thanks to better muscle tone and a reduction in body fat.

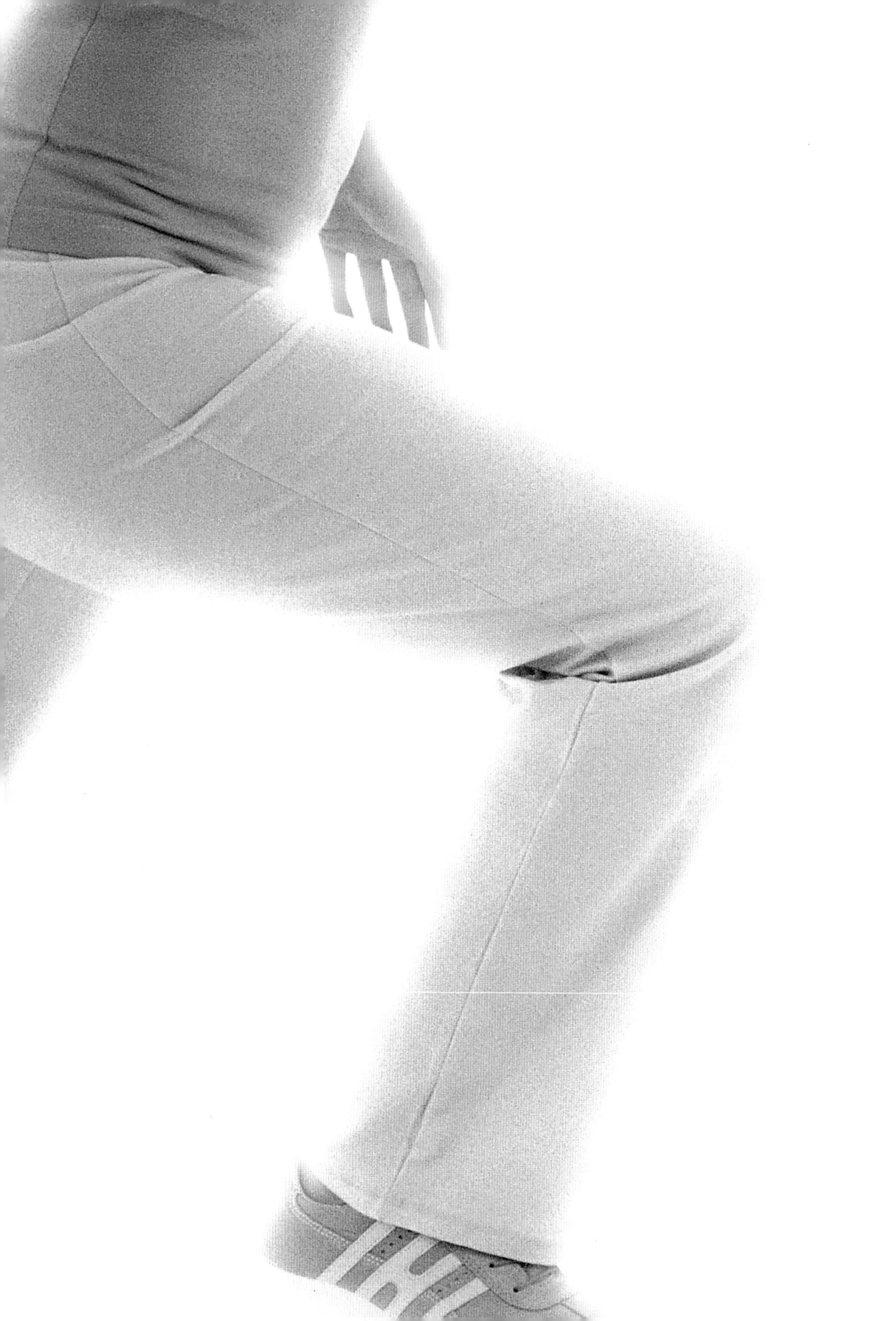

body sculpting basics

Why exercise?

One of the first steps towards sculpting a new body shape is to develop a regular exercise programme.

For a fit and healthy body we should be physically active always, right the way from childhood through to old age – be it 70, 80 or 90! Men and women who have exercised regularly throughout their lives have better muscle tone, strength and endurance, and therefore better overall quality of life than those who have not. This is because exercising helps maintain all the body's systems. All activities use energy; the more vigorous the activity the more calories you use. You obtain your energy through the food you eat. If you're active then you 'burn' the calories you've consumed as food; but if you eat too much food or do too little exercise the excess calories will be stored by your body as fat for use later. As you move your frame, muscles pull on bones and in doing so strengthen muscles, bones and the connective elements of tendons and ligaments in the process.

Learning new exercise routines or repeating old ones uses your brain and movement-to-mind paths, thereby keeping the mind alert, too. All this explains why your body will serve you better if you keep it in tip-top shape.

A regular routine

For good general health and a trim physique you'll need to include medium-intensity exercise in your life. Athletes or top-level competitors know what it is like to push their bodies to the limit. Most of us, however, have neither the time nor the inclination to push ourselves that far and, in fact, we don't need to. We simply need regular medium-paced exercise to maintain a healthy lifestyle that we can enjoy.

In the same way that we routinely brush our teeth each night or comb our hair in the morning, a certain level of exercise should become part of our routine to maintain our physical health. Start to think of exercise as something to be fitted in several times a week among all your other myriad routine tasks and it will become a natural part of your life. An exercise routine does not have to be very long. Thirty minutes will make a difference; an hour if you have it from week to week is great, but if you don't have an hour just make sure you do *something!*

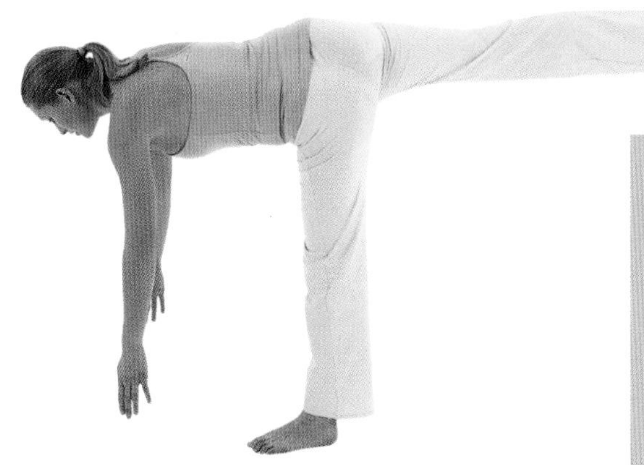

Change your body shape

As well as experiencing the holistic benefits of exercise you can improve your body shape (see page 26). There are many misconceptions about what makes up a good body and how you get one. Genetics, of course, play a large part in the kind of shape you have and the strengths and weaknesses of your body, including length of limbs and torso, basic bone frame and tendency towards fat or muscle. These things you cannot change. What you *can* change is the appearance of your body by assuming control over your body's amount of body fat and muscle.

Muscles lay over the bones and fat lays over and in between muscle (plus some fat is required internally for cushioning organs), providing the final layering that makes up your total shape. The amount of body fat you have is dictated by the quantity and type of food you consume and by how many calories you burn off throughout the day. How much muscle mass you have is dictated by what you use your body for. If it needs more muscle then your body builds it. If your body is underused then muscle can waste away. Body sculpting is the path to changing your muscle mass or body fat ratio. Contrary to popular belief, fat does not turn into muscle, nor muscle into fat.

Benefits of regular exercise

- **You will reduce the risk of diseases** such as heart disease and cancer and conditions like high blood pressure and osteoporosis
- **Cholesterol levels** in the blood are better controlled
- **Feeling refreshed** and **less stressed** are immediate results of exercise; regular exercise is a great stress-buster
- **Better eating and drinking habits** will develop as you become more interested in and aware of your body and start to look after it better. Your body also starts to crave the 'right' kind of foods
- **Weight control** can be helped by aerobic exercise, such as jogging or skipping, that uses stored fat to maintain energy levels
- **A good-looking body** gives you more confidence and increased *joie de vivre*
- **Exercise-induced sweating** and thirst will encourage the replacement of lost fluids. Drinking water regularly helps the body systems and keeps the bladder healthy
- **Your mood** and **feelings of wellbeing** will be boosted by exercise, which can help ward off depression
- **Mind-to-movement paths** are improved – you'll feel more coordinated and in control

Body sculpting explained

Body sculpting essentially involves cardiovascular (CV) exercise to burn excess body fat, muscle-building, or toning, to give you a streamlined appearance, and stretching to lengthen muscles after exercise and to aid your flexibility.

How muscles work

To sculpt your body into an improved shape, you need to appreciate how muscles work. When you exercise – or perform any activity – impulses sent from the brain cause contraction, or shortening, in the muscles, which pull on bones via tendons and ligaments to move the limbs and torso. As you contract the muscles you work them and thereby maintain their form. If you start to work your muscles more forcefully, for example by contracting them against resistance, the muscles will start to become stronger, which emphasizes the tone of the muscle but not, greatly, its size. By working your muscles you can start to create, or sculpt, a new shape for yourself.

Women are often anxious not to build muscle, frightened they may end up looking masculine or bulky. The reality is that most women would need to do an Olympic-style training programme and radically change their diet to gain huge muscle mass. Added muscle tone simply gives you greater strength and a more defined and sculpted shape.

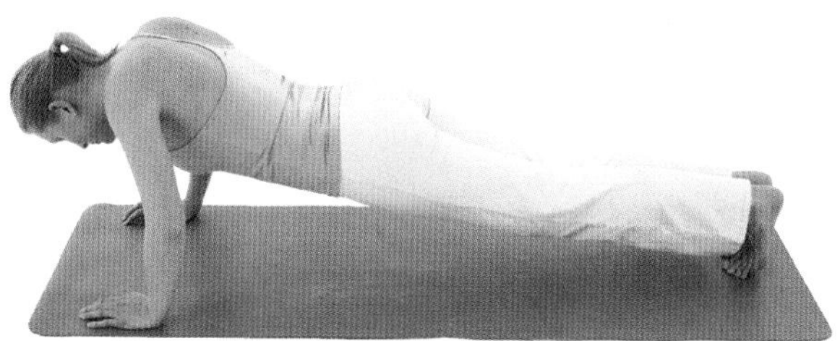

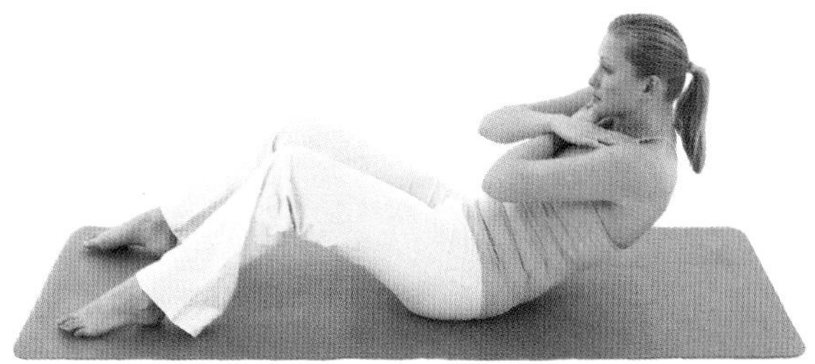

Which muscles are you working?

In fitness moves and in normal everyday movement it is rarely one muscle alone doing all the work. Most movements are a combination of many muscles working cooperatively. Some muscles may be maintaining your posture as you perform the move – these are referred to as the stabilizers. Other muscles may be assisting the movement. If just one muscle is doing the bulk of the work, it is called the prime mover. Sometimes you can even get one set of muscles to work against another in order to enhance the muscle resistance or the stretch (see page 125).

If you are unsure which muscles you are working in a particular exercise, just remember that muscles work by contraction. So when you perform an exercise look carefully at your body and notice which muscle is contracting (shortening) and note where you can feel the effort of the contraction.

Benefits of good muscle tone

- Increased strength in the heart, lungs and muscles, thereby keeping them healthy
- Increased overall energy
- Improved posture and appearance
- Prevention of injury and degeneration
- Better weight control since larger muscles use up more calories
- Good posture and stability resulting in improved flexibility
- Good muscle tone goes hand-in-hand with stronger bones, helping slow down the normal ageing process of bone loss, which occurs in adults from their mid-30s

Using resistance to build muscle

Muscle fibres are built by contracting the 'belly' of the muscle. A workout that involves contracting the muscles against a resistance means that when the muscle contracts while pulling or pushing against a load, it has to work harder than normal. After the workout the muscle repairs itself by building new fibres to become stronger and cope with the extra demand. This is your goal with the body-sculpting programme. You will be doing exercises that gently stress and overload your muscles so that they become stronger and more defined in shape. The other key element of body sculpting involves stretching out and maintaining length in your muscles as you build (see page 18).

There are numerous ways to provide resistance (see page 16). Your own body weight can provide resistance as you move, for example when doing press-ups (see page 99). As you lower your straight body down via your arms, your arm muscles are working to lower the body with control. Without their muscular resistance your body would just crash to the ground. If your body does collapse into the floor when you first attempt a press-up it is because your muscles are not yet strong enough. It can take up to six weeks of regular practice (working out three or four times per week) for muscles to gain in strength and therefore shape.

Another way of adding further resistance to moving muscles is by using weights during a workout (see page 16) to improve your strength even faster.

Build up gradually

Note that when working with weights or your own body weight, you need to build up gradually. When muscles are challenged they will take a couple of days to repair. If you stress your muscles too much too soon you will experience painful stiffness. The exact mechanisms of stiffness are still unknown. Researchers believe that when you overwork muscles unaccustomed to the level of stress, you cause microscopic tears in the muscle; as these tears repair, the muscle itself feels stiff. Within two or three days, however, this discomfort will pass and the muscles will have rebuilt themselves more strongly.

Muscle map

These diagrams will show you where your muscles are. You may well find it helps your training if you visualize which muscles you are working.

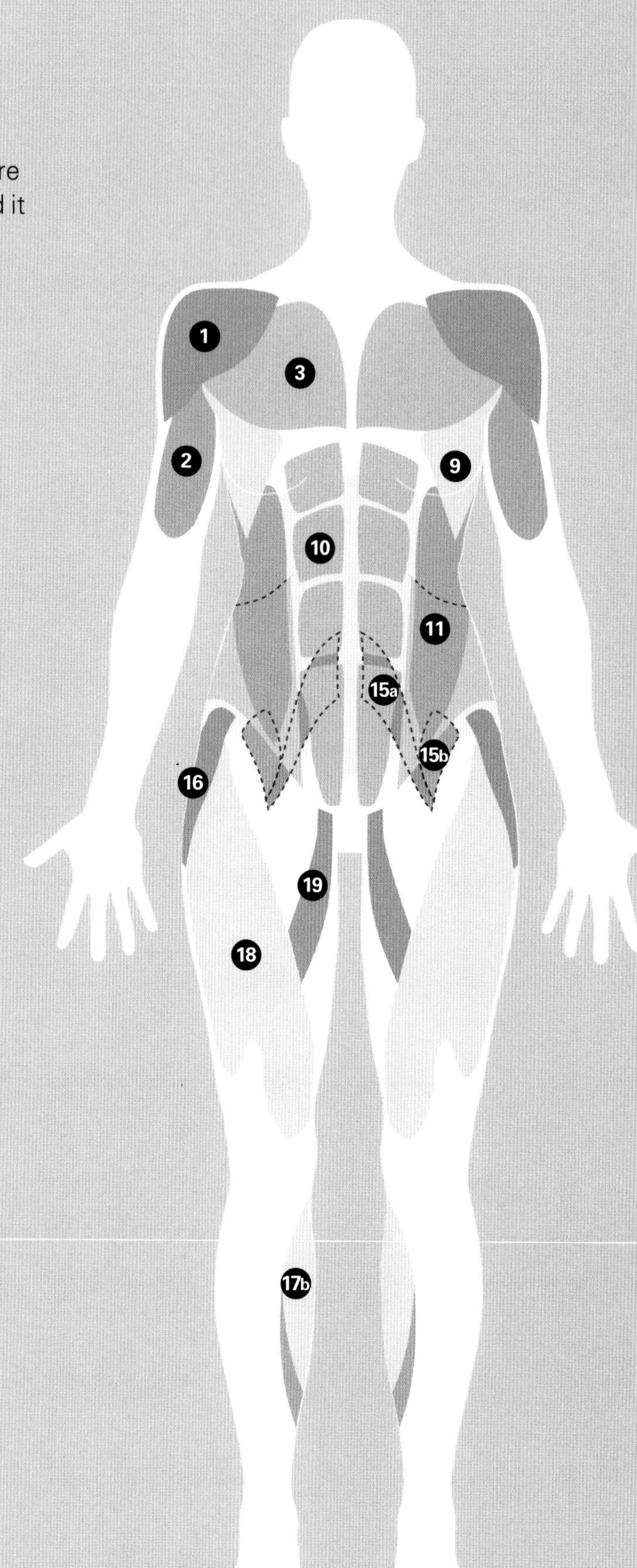

Muscle names

1 **Deltoids** (shoulder)
2 **Biceps** (front of upper arms)
3 **Pectoralis major** (chest muscles)
4 **Triceps** (back of upper arms)
5 **Rhomboids** (muscles between shoulder blades)
6 **Trapezius** (upper back muscles)
7 **Posterior deltoids** (rear of shoulder)
8 **Infraspinatus** (middle back muscles)
9 **Serratus anterior (upper ribcage muscle)**
10 **Rectus abdominis** (front abdominal muscle)
11 **Abdominal muscles:**

External obliques (side abdominal muscles – these run down the sides of your torso between the chest and the pelvis)

Internal obliques (side abdominal muscles – these lie beneath the external obliques, connecting the last four ribs with the pelvis)

Transversus abdominis (inner abdominal muscle – this lies underneath the rectus abdominis)

12 **Pelvic floor muscles** (not shown – these are the muscles between your legs that form the base of the pelvic basin. They support your internal organs)
13 **Gluteus medius** (buttock muscle)
14 **Gluteus maximus** (buttock muscle)
15a **Psoas major** (hip flexor)
15b **Iliacus** (hip flexor)
16 **Tensor fasciae latae** (outer thigh muscle)
17a **Gastrocnemius** (calf muscle)
17b **Soleus** (calf muscle)
18 **Quadriceps** (front thigh muscles)
19 **Adductor longus** (inner thigh muscle)
20 **Biceps femoris, semitendonosus and semimembranosus** (hamstrings)

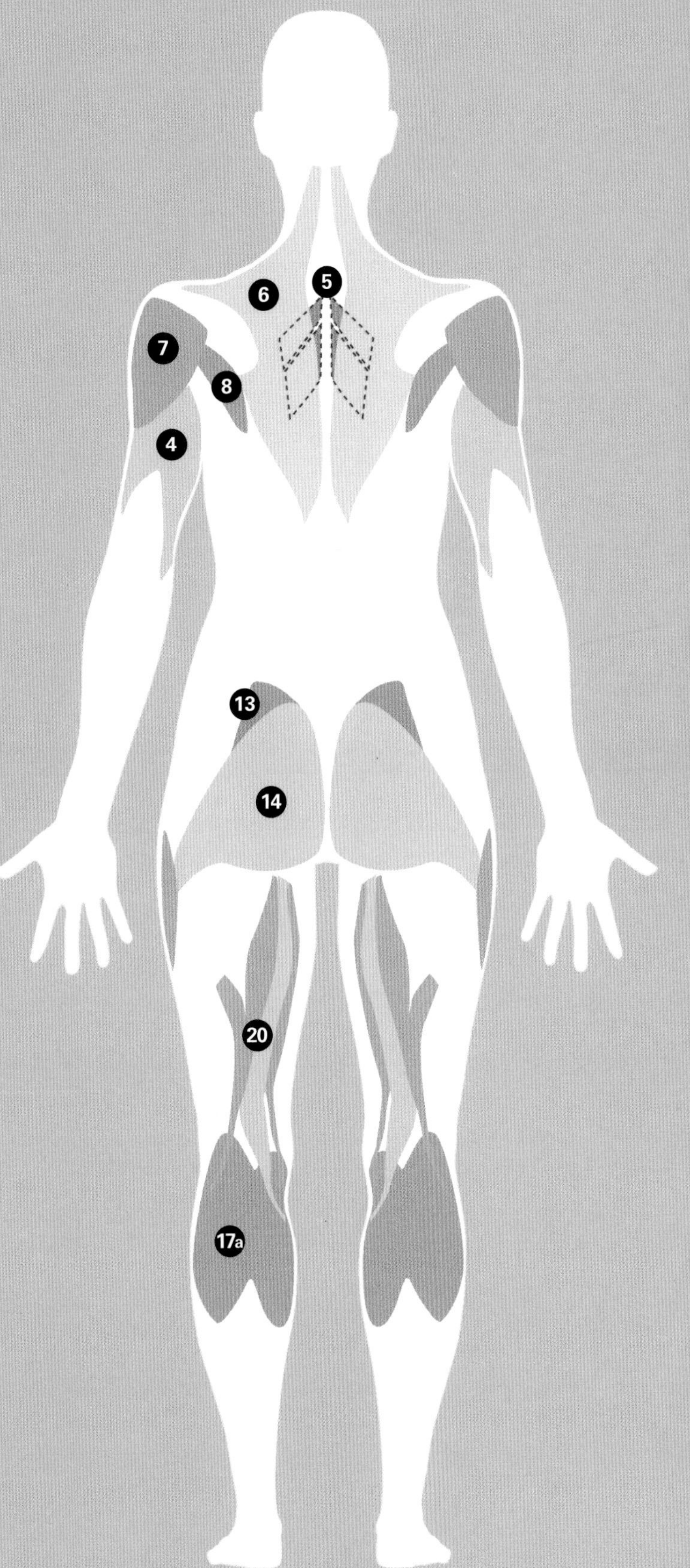

Different ways of toning

You now know that to tone muscles effectively you have to work them against resistance. As with stretching (see page 18), there are a number of different ways to do this. The types of toning work featured in your six-week programme concentrate on the first two listed below – body building (as defined here) and weight training. These two methods allow you to focus on specific body areas and to develop the muscles in these areas as part of your body-sculpting programme.

Working with your body weight

The real meaning of body building is to exercise using your own body weight to increase muscle mass.

- **Press-ups** This is a good example of using your weight to exercise your arms (see page 99).
- **Sit-ups** When you take your weight on to your back and curl your head and shoulders off the floor to perform a sit-up, you are toning the abdominals as they work to contract against the weight of your upper body.
- **Swiss ball** This large, inflated ball is used for fitness training and allows the body to work in positions that are even more challenging.

Working with weights

Another way to stress and tone muscles is to use weights. By lifting a weight you add extra resistance to the natural muscle movement so your muscles have to work that much harder. The heavier the weight you lift or push, the harder your muscles – and the rest of the body in support – has to work.

The benefit of weights like dumbbells (a hand-held weight) and barbells (a long pole with weights at either end) is that you can load up the weights so that the workload is greater and the benefits come sooner. Other kinds of resistance equipment, including weighted balls, resistance bands and abdominizers, all help to tone the muscles.

Working your heart and lungs

All sporting activities will tone the muscles. As you run, jump, catch and throw you are naturally stressing and toning the muscles. The more vigorous and intense the sport, the more intense the contractions of the muscles.

Although not conventionally referred to as toning, cardiovascular (CV) exercise does have a toning quality that is important to remember. CV exercise is generally regarded as aerobic – meaning that oxygen is used in the body to break down fat into energy to keep the body going. CV exercise essentially works the heart and lungs and therefore tones these areas. When you run, walk, jump, skip and jog energetically for any extended period of time (at least 10 minutes) you are stressing the heart muscle, requiring it to pump harder and faster to meet the extra demands made of it. When you do this regularly, the heart muscle, like all muscles, responds by becoming stronger and larger. As you exercise the lungs, they also become more efficient in supplying oxygen to the muscles and other body systems much quicker.

Toning postural muscles

An important set of muscles that require toning are the postural muscles. These are hard to define, but can be described as all the smaller muscles along the frame that assist the movements of the larger muscles.

1 When you perform an exercise there tends to be one major muscle that is doing most of the work – this is called the prime mover. For instance, when you perform a triceps extension, the prime mover could be identified as the triceps muscle. However, there are many other muscles working at the same time during this exercise – muscles to support the position of the arms, muscles in the stomach keeping the torso straight and muscles in the legs and feet maintaining your balance. These smaller muscles are used every time you perform a movement, be it large or small.

2 Whenever you do an exercise where balance and alignment come into play you make the postural muscles work hard. When you use a Swiss ball to sit on and perform upper body exercises, for example, you work the postural muscles of the torso and hips to maintain your balance and position on the ball.

3 When you perform movements on one leg, such as the arabesque movement of a ballet class, you are working not only the muscles of the buttock to lift and hold the leg, but also the muscles of the supporting leg and foot to adjust and balance the full weight of the body on one foot.

When you perform these kinds of exercises regularly you will notice a greater freedom and control of movement in everyday life.

It is important to check your body's alignment and general posture before starting a workout programme (see page 28) so that you can assess whether there are any problems that need sorting out before you start.

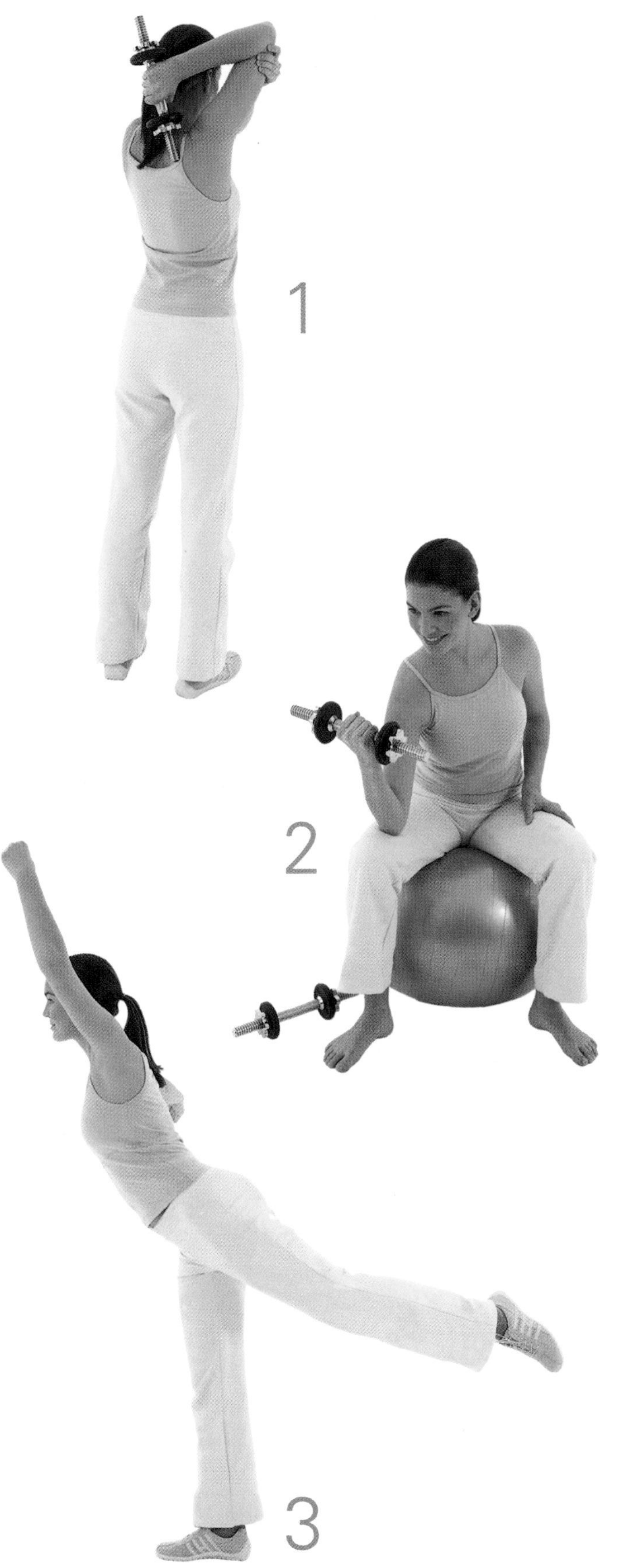

The importance of stretching

The opposite of muscle toning is stretching. Toning involves contracting the muscle whereas stretching involves lengthening it; stretching is just as important to body sculpting as toning. When you contract and release muscles you are shortening the muscle fibres to produce movement. When you perform these movements against substantial resistance the muscles are contracting regularly and forcefully. At the end of a workout it is therefore essential to rebalance your body by lengthening the contracted muscles via stretching exercises.

What does stretching involve?

Stretching simply places limbs in such a position that the muscle is extended and maintaining its length for some seconds to allow it to return to normal. Although stretching does not influence the size and strength of the muscle, it can influence its shape – which is why stretching has an equally important role within body sculpting.

As you build and strengthen muscle you need to keep it as mobile and as long as you can. Stretching out the muscles each time after muscle toning takes little effort and will ensure the muscle fibres are lengthened as they build. This will contribute to your overall streamlined shape, as well as your mobility and balance.

If you overtrain on the toning side without putting in the work on the stretching side you can create problems for yourself as overcontracted muscles are more prone to injury from tearing and snapping. Similarly, problems can also be encountered by body builders who overtrain and pump up their muscles, often losing flexibility and ease of movement in the process.

Preventing injury

To feel really fit and able on a day-to-day basis you should be aiming to do regular – and, importantly, varied – exercise. The problem with some sports and activities is that they can start to tighten certain muscles. CV exercise, for example, is an important element of fitness but tends to focus on the leg muscles for running and jumping. The leg muscles, particularly the back of the legs, can start to tighten up significantly with such constant work. This is why people who run regularly, play football, tennis or squash can all be prone to tight hamstrings and calf muscles. This can cause problems with the Achilles tendon at the back of the heel, as tight calves pull on the tendon. Similarly, tight hamstrings can cause problems by stressing the back.

Stretching out regularly therefore becomes a very important element of your body-sculpting programme – not only for 'all roundness' but also for injury prevention.

Different ways of stretching

The three basic stretches are active, passive and developmental, all of which will stand you in good stead when it comes to body sculpting. Most of the warm-up moves and the cool-down stretches in the six-week programmes in this book use these types of stretches. Stretching has been used as part of the warm-up in fitness routines for some decades now. Remember, however, that the muscles need to be warm to be stretched safely (see box, below). Stretching has a place in warming up but only as a brief portion of the warm-up and the best stretches to do are active ones.

1 Active stretch

You perform a stretch when you actively move one muscle group while naturally stretching another. A high forward kick is an example. As your quadriceps muscles contract to extend and lift the leg, the hamstrings at the back of the thigh are forced to stretch a little.

This type of stretch is momentary and not held for any length of time. It lengthens the muscle under gentle force and allows the body to keep moving. This not only keeps the body warm but also allows the body to rehearse some of the moves it might make later during the more intense section of the workout. This rehearsal and building of body heat helps keep you injury-free as you work out.

Warming up before stretching

One of the most important things to remember before you begin any kind of stretching is that you should be warm. When you raise the body's core temperature the synovial fluid between the joints is warmed and inclined to allow the surfaces to pass more freely over one another. The blood flow is increased and the muscles are warmed as you keep moving, so the body moves much more freely and your potential for stretching to your limits is increased. There are various ways to warm up before stretching:

- Exercise using your arms and legs until you sweat
- Go for a gentle run or cycle
- Use a rowing machine or dance to your favourite music for 15 minutes
- Work out for at least 20 minutes so that you are warm
- Sit in a sauna for 15 minutes

The essence of body sculpting

The combination of toning and stretching, with some CV work is the key to sculpting your body, that is changing your muscle mass or body fat ratio.

- As you work your muscles against resistance you build more muscle fibres
- More muscle fibres will give you stronger muscles and a more defined shape
- Increased muscle mass means more calorie-demanding fibres, so instead of extra calories being stored as fat they are used up by your muscles
- Stretching keeps the muscles you are building lengthened and sleek
- Stretching also keeps you mobile and flexible thereby helping to prevent injury

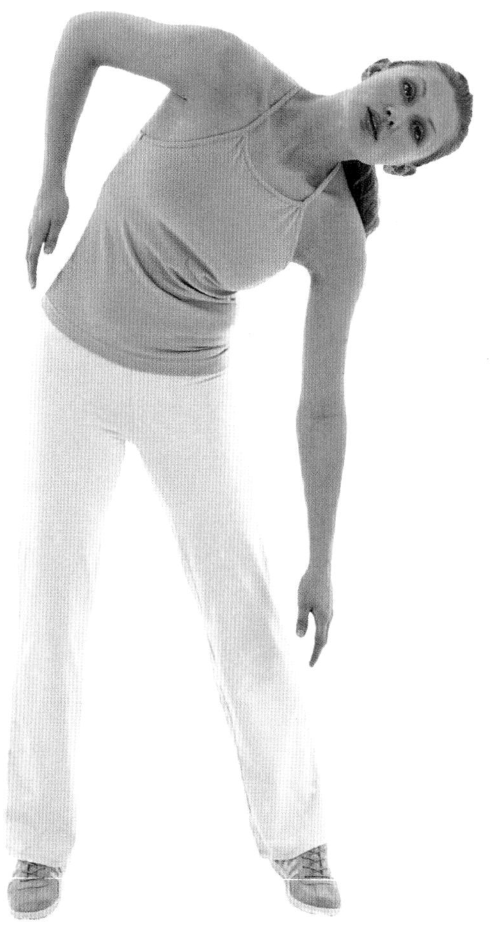

2 Passive stretch

This type of stretch is one where the muscles are relaxed – you allow the weight of your body (in certain positions) to pull you further into the stretch. Passive stretches should be done only when the body is thoroughly warmed up.

Many workout videos feature a stretching session immediately after the warm-up; however, it is debatable as to how beneficial this is. If you have performed some active stretches like kicks, side bends and lunges during your warm-up, the chances are your body will be stretched enough to continue the rest of the workout. Stopping to perform lengthy passive stretches at this point will only cool your body's core temperature and lead to your overall energy being lowered. Passive stretches are best performed at the end of the routine or briefly during the session as a counterbalance to the previous move.

3 Developmental stretch

Developmental stretches improve your flexibility. They involve taking the stretch to the point where you feel you are at your natural limit and then trying to take it a little further (see page 124).

Stretching for relaxation

Stretching for relaxation may seem like an oxymoron but gentle stretching of stiff or tired muscles can actually be very relaxing to both the mind and the body. Although stretching and mobilizing are active things, certain stretches allow you to rest in these positions and let your mind wander as your body starts to relax. Relaxation stretches are not so much for developing flexibility but for helping you become at ease with your body. The following gentle stretch is an example.

▲ Child pose

1 Kneel on the floor, with your bottom sitting on your heels. Lean forward and rest your forehead on the floor, at the same time stretching your arms out straight in front of you. Let your body sink into the position as you breathe normally.

2 As you maintain this position you should feel your body start to make minor adjustments. You will feel the weight of your head pressing further into the floor as your neck muscles relax. You will feel a release in your shoulders as you relax your elbows on to the floor. You may feel your lower back release as your bottom sinks on to your heels. All these things happen not because you are pushing the body into these positions, but because you are staying in a position long enough for the body to make its own adjustments.

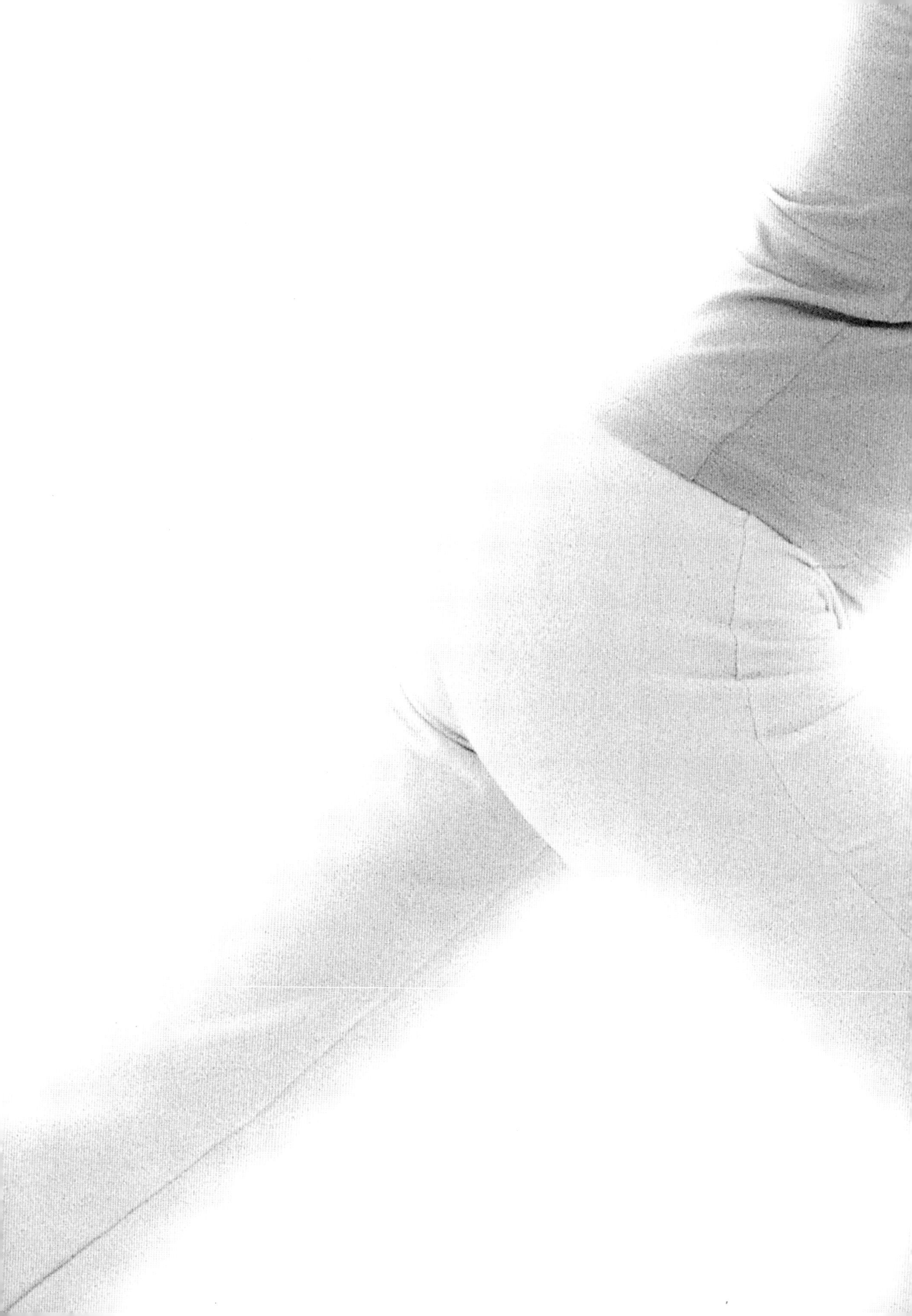

assessing your shape

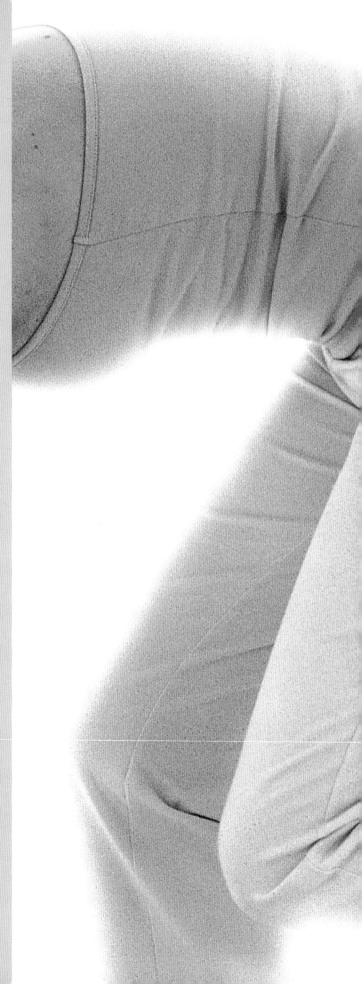

Assess yourself

One of the most important things to do before you start one of the six-week programmes is to decide what you really want to get out of it. The following pages will help you take a good long look at your shape, your body and your capabilities in order to see how to approach your programme. Aim to identify key areas that you wish to improve, then you can pick and choose from each six-week programme accordingly.

You will have a clear idea of how to approach the next six weeks if you first work your way through the following assessments:

- body type
- posture
- fitness levels
- body fat

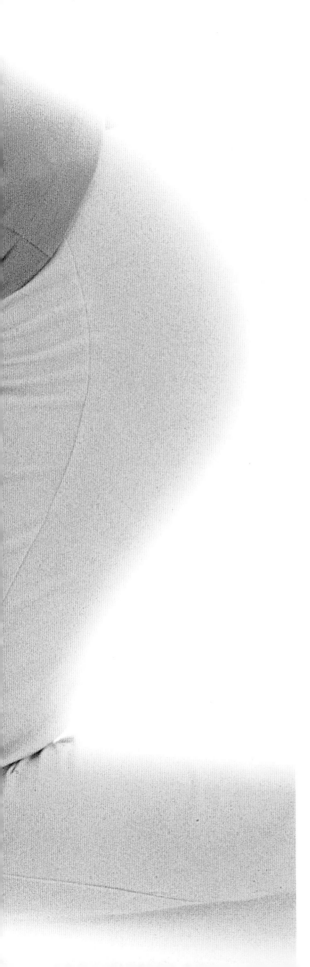

Assessing your body type

There are various ways to define body type, and you will probably already have a good idea of your own body type. Some people say things like: 'I only have to look at a cream cake and I put on weight'. Another person might say: 'If I lift any kind of weights I put on too much muscle'. What they are defining, probably without realizing it, are the natural tendencies of their own body (see page 26).

Our tendencies towards different types of musculature and physicality – and even our preference for different types of exercise – may all be passed down in our genes. They are then shaped further by our personalities. This is worth taking into account when you plan your workouts as it can affect what type of exercise programme you will enjoy and be able to stick to.

Different people enjoy different things

Most people tend to enjoy the types of exercise they are good at – and find relatively easy. If there is an exercise you find hard then this is the exercise you tend to avoid. In the same way, different people feel pain in different ways. Some people are able to undergo and even enjoy the breathlessness of a hard run, while for others this feeling can panic them. Other people prefer to tire their muscles with weights – they will feel 'the burn' in their muscles and they will enjoy the struggle of the last repetition. Still other people enjoy the feeling of stretching their muscles – maintaining a stretch position is both relaxing and pleasurable – whereas for others the stretching sensation can be nearer agony.

So the type of exercise you enjoy can tell you a lot about your body type and the way your body prefers to move. People who enjoy endurance sports tend to have longer, leaner and less pronounced muscles, while people who enjoy heavy lifting-type sports tend to have clearer defined muscles. Our bodies reflect very accurately what we do.

Body types

Dr William H Sheldon, working in the 1940s, first introduced the notion of somatypes, which puts body types into three categories – ectomorph, mesomorph and endomorph. Look at the following definitions and you should be able to identify yourself as one of these body types. Once you have an idea of your body type, move on to take a look at your posture (see page 28).

Ectomorph

This body type tends to be thinner and more fragile than the other types, with a delicate or lightly muscled frame. Ectomorphs tend to be taller and can even be stoop-shouldered.

- **Muscle growth in this type takes longer.**

Weakness

If this is your type then you will find it harder to build muscle and you will probably feel less inclined to do toning exercises.

Solution

You should aim to do some toning, however, because it helps keep the skeleton supported and using muscles is important for keeping the bones strong. Doing more repetitions with lighter weights or doing more choreographed toning to music might well help your enjoyment of this kind of exercise.

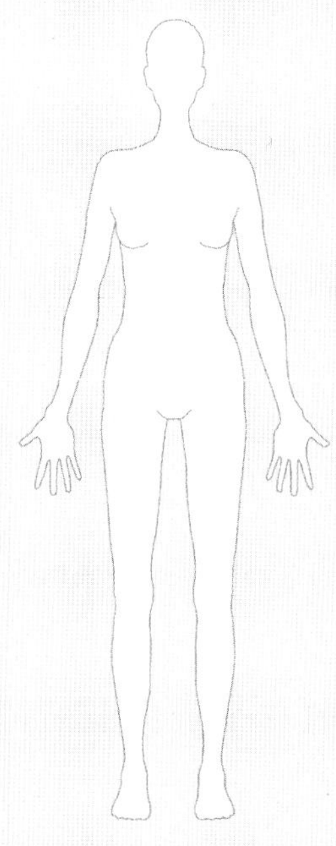

Mesomorph

This body type tends to be athletic-looking with a harder muscular appearance. Some female mesomorphs can be rectangular or hourglass-shaped with a thicker skin and upright posture.

• This body type grows muscle quickly and can usually lose – and gain – weight easily.

Weakness

If this is your type, toning up may happen fairly quickly but you may lack flexibility. You may also feel less inclined to do CV exercises.

Solution

You need to focus on the stretching side of the body sculpting programme to ensure that your musculature isn't compromised by lack of flexibility. Don't forget CV exercises in your training either, as it is important to get your heart pumping on a regular basis to keep your heart and CV system in good shape.

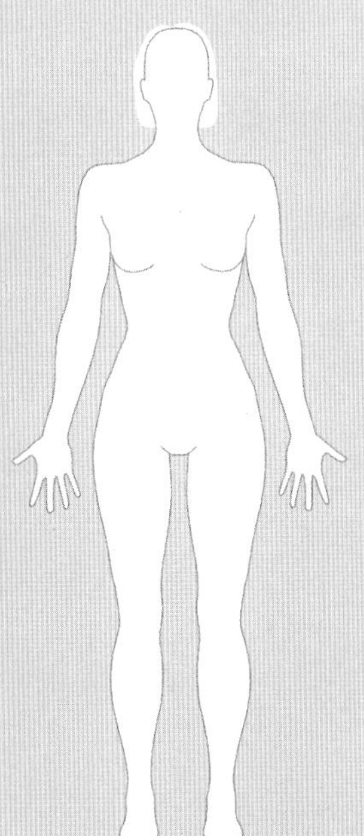

Endomorph

This body type tends towards a soft body that can be flabby. Muscles tend to be under-developed and the shape rounded.

• It is usually harder for endomorphs to lose weight but they can gain muscle relatively easily.

Weakness

If you feel this is your type then you will need to be disciplined about putting in some hard work on muscle-building. You may find this kind of exercise tougher than other types but keep in mind that it will really help improve your shape.

Solution

Muscle is smoother-looking and harder than fat so more muscle will actually streamline your appearance. You need to work consistently to build the muscle – it will take six to eight weeks to build new muscle tissue if you work out twice a week (results will be quicker with more workouts each week).

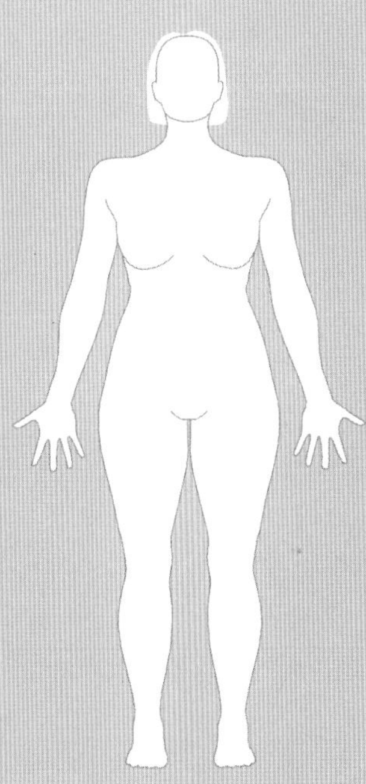

Assessing your posture

The following test will draw your attention to your natural way of sitting and standing. If your posture is poor and you are allowing your body to sag, then many of your smaller muscles are not being used. To do this test properly, you ideally need two long mirrors – one in front of you and the other placed, at an angle, just behind you. Stand in front of the mirror so that you have a front and a back view of your full body. Wear only your underwear so that you can clearly see your waist, knees and hips. Observe your standing position then answer the questions below.

Looking at yourself from the front:

1. Is your **head** held erect, neither tilted to the left nor to the right? ☐ Yes ☐ No
2. Are both **shoulders** the same height above the floor? ☐ Yes ☐ No
3. When your **hands** are outstretched, are the tips of the **longest fingers** on each hand the same distance from the floor? ☐ Yes ☐ No
4. Are your **hip bones** the same height above the floor? ☐ Yes ☐ No
5. Are your **kneecaps** the same height above the floor and do they appear to be facing forwards? ☐ Yes ☐ No
6. Is your body weight resting on the centre of each **foot** rather than on the inner borders of the feet? ☐ Yes ☐ No

Looking at yourself from the back:

7. Are your **shoulder blades** the same height above the floor and do they protrude from the back of your ribcage? ☐ Yes ☐ No
8. Is your **backbone** (the spines of the vertebrae) in a vertical straight line? ☐ Yes ☐ No
9. Is there an equal gap between your **elbows** and your **hips** on each side? ☐ Yes ☐ No

Take a good look at the back of your lower legs and heels:

10. Does the **Achilles tendon** seem to be going straight up each calf from the ankle? ☐ Yes ☐ No

Now stand sideways on and observe your stance:

11. Is your **head** held erect, the **chin** neither pulled back nor jutting out? ☐ Yes ☐ No
12. Are your **shoulders** upright, rather than rounded? ☐ Yes ☐ No
13. Is the curvature of your **lower back** gentle rather than severely arched, and your **ribs** not protruding? ☐ Yes ☐ No
14. Are your **lower legs** aligned with the **thighs** and the **knees** and not pushed backwards (hyperextended)? ☐ Yes ☐ No

Interpreting the results

People with poor posture inevitably have some muscles that are short and tight while other muscles are elongated and often relatively weak. Some of the most common things you may notice include rounded shoulders, an arched lower back or hyperextended knees.

• Questions 1–4

If you answered 'no' to one or more statements, you might have some degree of scoliosis, or a side-to-side curvature of the spine. This could cause discomfort and even injury during vigorous exercise. If this is very pronounced you should consult a general practitioner or registered osteopath before you begin your body sculpting programme.

• Question 5

If you answered 'no' you may have a condition known as 'squinting patella', for which you should consult a registered osteopath. You should also pay great attention to pulling up in your thighs when you stand and check that your knees are in line with the toes each time you bend your knees.

• Question 6

A 'no' answer may mean you have a condition known as 'excessive pronation' or 'over pronation', which is caused by excessive flexibility in the joints of the foot and the collapse of the arches of the feet. The condition is very common and may lead to painful disorders of the knee joints and discomfort in the shins. Your body weight should be distributed evenly on the feet. Over-emphasis on the outer or inner borders (supination/pronation) can lead to problems with the ankles and Achilles tendons. Always check you are balancing on the middle of your feet. Check, as you begin each exercise, that you are not allowing your ankles to fall out or in.

• Question 7

A 'no' answer here may mean you are suffering from a condition known as 'winged scapulae' a weakness of the muscles under the shoulder blades and a tightness of the muscles of the chest region. Look for stretches for the chest in the six-week programmes and make sure you do these regularly, continuing them after the six weeks.

• Question 8

A 'no' answer to this question may also indicate scoliosis of the spine (see answer to questions 1–4).

• Question 9

If you have answered 'no', it may indicate your pelvis is out of alignment, with a tendency for your hips to twist. Stretching out the sides of the body as much as possible will help with this, as will a visit to a registered osteopath.

• Question 10

If you have answered 'no', you may have a bowed Achilles tendon which can indicate incorrect foot positions and may lead to Achilles problems. Check you are not rolling in or out on your feet.

• Questions 11–13

If you have checked 'no' for any of these items, it strongly indicates slouched posture. Always try to be aware of lifting 'up and out' of the top of your head when you stand. Feel as though the top of your head is pressing to the ceiling. As you work your way through the six-week programmes you will become stronger and more supple and this will start to reverse any slouching.

• Question 14

Hyperextended knees are very common and can lead to bad posture further up the spine. Always stand with your thighs pulled up, which lifts the kneecaps. This will stop you pressing back on the back of your knees, which can damage the ligaments.

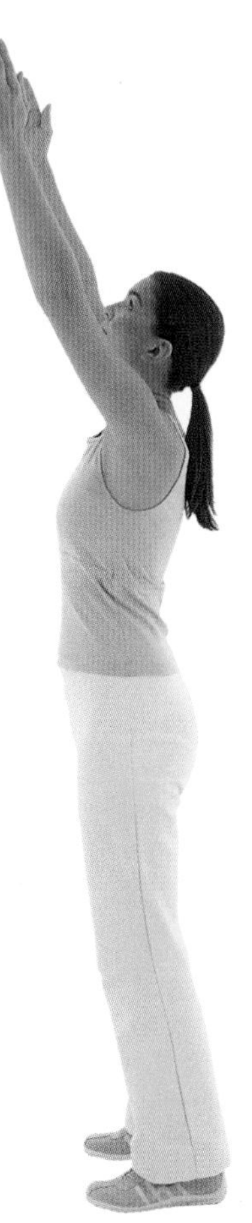

Assessing your fitness levels

The final assessment to make before beginning your body-sculpting programme is to think about yourself and how you feel at the moment. Answer the questions below to get a complete picture. When you have looked at the results, keep a note of the body area you feel you need to work on first.

A

1. Do you feel fit? ☐ Yes ☐ No
2. Can you move around easily? ☐ Yes ☐ No
3. Can you touch your toes and put your socks on easily? ☐ Yes ☐ No
4. Can you kick your legs up in the air if you need to? ☐ Yes ☐ No
5. Do you feel you can twist and turn easily? ☐ Yes ☐ No
6. Do you wake up in the morning not feeling stiff? ☐ Yes ☐ No
7. Can you move without pain or tweaks and groans? ☐ Yes ☐ No

B

8. Do you feel strong? ☐ Yes ☐ No
9. Could you move a large armchair by yourself if you had to? ☐ Yes ☐ No
10. Can you bend with all your weight on one leg and get up again? ☐ Yes ☐ No
11. Can you put one foot on to a slightly higher stool and lift your body weight up on to it? ☐ Yes ☐ No
12. Can you lift several heavy shopping bags? ☐ Yes ☐ No
13. Do you feel lively most of the time? ☐ Yes ☐ No
14. Can you perform unexpected movements without pulling something or being dreadfully stiff the next day? ☐ Yes ☐ No

15. Do you feel energetic most of the time? ☐ Yes ☐ No
16. Do you generally feel positive? ☐ Yes ☐ No
17. Are you sleeping well? ☐ Yes ☐ No
18. Are you happy with how your body looks at the moment? ☐ Yes ☐ No
19. Do you like yourself generally at the moment? ☐ Yes ☐ No
20. Is your confidence level good at the moment? ☐ Yes ☐ No
21. Are you happy with your sexual relationship at the moment? ☐ Yes ☐ No
22. Is there more than one area of your body that you are happy with? ☐ Yes ☐ No

Interpreting the results

Working out which areas of fitness you need to concentrate on will help you really focus on your programme. The results will identify which areas may be your weakest.

A

If you answered 'no' to most of questions 1–7 you are probably feeling a little unfit in the flexibility department. This is an important aspect of overall fitness as it is something that really affects our daily life. As we get older, from our mid-30s onwards, the body tends to become stiffer; muscles tend to tighten and shorten if they are not specifically worked on to maintain their length. When you do your six-week programmes, focus on all the stretching exercises and keep them as a constant theme throughout your workouts so that you can really start to limber up again. Whatever age you are, once you start doing some flexibility exercises on a regular basis, you will notice an increase in mobility and enhanced freedom of movement.

B

If you answered 'no' to most of questions 8–14 what is bothering you most about your fitness is your lack of muscle tone. Muscles move our body and protect our frame. Without strong postural muscles the body will make compensations, and aches and injuries can occur. If some of the basic muscles are weak then it is hard to perform even basic everyday tasks easily and safely. As you build strong muscle fibre you will find your body will do what you ask of it more easily and your confidence will increase tenfold.

C

If you answered 'no' to most of questions 15–22 you are probably suffering from a lack of cardiovascular fitness and an excess of stress. Stress can affect our sleeping, confidence and general outlook on life. One of the best ways to combat stress is regular exercise. When you exercise you are focusing on something other than yourself. You should be thinking about the moves you are doing and how to do them more effectively. In this way your mind gets a break from thinking about your daily tasks. CV exercise will improve the performance of your heart and lungs, and this will also increase your ability to deal with stress.

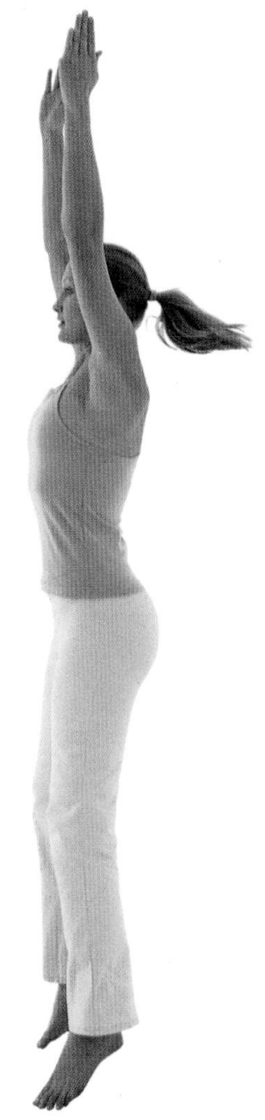

Body fat

You should by now be able to figure out what is lacking in your fitness regime and what you need to do about it. You may also be aware that you have some excess body fat to lose, although the constant pressure that we are put under by a weight-obsessed society shouldn't be your reason for wanting to lose weight. However, it is a basic health issue that you should remain within certain weight ranges. More and more scientific studies prove that being excessively overweight can increase the risk of many diseases, illnesses and problems, ranging from diabetes and cancer to back pain and snoring.

Be realistic

A basic issue when tackling excess weight is to first make sure that you are not aiming to fix what is wrong in your life by trying to change your body. If you are unhappy with your marriage or your job, for example, these problems will not be solved simply by losing weight. Also, be aware that many photographs of models are 'touched up' for publication. The camera *can* lie these days so don't believe everything you see and don't model your body on someone else's!

Don't be fooled

Because losing weight has become such a hot topic over the years, there are many myths about the body and how it works. But don't be fooled! To approach a weight-loss programme realistically, you must understand that there are no shortcuts. Once you have gained weight, it can (without hard work) be a very long process to get rid of it.

For most people, gaining weight is a slow process – the result of taking in too much energy (in the form of food) gradually over some years. Being the efficient survival mechanism it is, the body stores excess energy for use at a later date.

Gaining weight actually takes exactly the same amount of time as losing it. The problem is that when we gain weight we are so busy with our lives we scarcely notice. Yet when we do notice we immediately want to rid ourselves of all that excess stored fat!

Guestimate

Ask yourself honestly...

- how long did it take you to gain the weight you now wish to lose?
- Did it creep on over the last four years?
- Have you been gaining weight since you left school?
- Did you just recently gain 5 kg (10½ lb)?

Your answer will tell you two things:

- What has caused you to put on weight, and therefore how to avoid putting on further weight in the future.
- How long it will take you to reverse the process.

Calculate the length of time it took you to gain the weight. Then work out one-quarter of this figure and, with *lots* of determination – and the aid of this book! – this is the length of time it will take you to lose it.

How exercise helps change your shape

The best shape you can be in is to be fit and healthy all over with strong musculature throughout the body and a low percentage of body fat. Muscles should be toned and flexible, allowing full range of movement, with no restriction due to body fat or tight joints. To get your best shape, you need to concentrate on CV conditioning, muscle-building work (toning) and flexibility work (stretching).

CV work plays its part

For each of the total 24 weeks depicted in this book you will find an exercise that focuses on CV conditioning and you should try to build up the length of time you perform such exercise. Whenever you exercise rhythmically and constantly, in excess of 15–20 minutes, the body uses oxygen to metabolize stored fat into energy to enable the body to keep going. Therefore by performing the CV exercises in this book for at least 15–20 minutes you will start to rid your frame of excess fat.

Toning takes its toll

When you perform toning exercises, the muscles and bones are stressed and respond by becoming stronger and leaner. One of the quickest ways to increase muscle mass is by working with resistance weight (see page 16).

Some of the routines in this book require you to use dumbbells, for which you first need to calculate how heavy a weight you should be lifting. If you lift weights that are too heavy you could overstress a muscle, ligament or tendon. If you lift weights that are too light, however, your results will be slow in showing. For safe but quick body-sculpting results you should be performing exercises made up of a safe but low number of repetitions – a set of 10 repetitions (known as reps for short) is advised (see page 34)

Keep mobile

The final piece of the fitness puzzle, once you have mastered the principles, is to ensure that you maintain your body's flexibility. As you gain muscle and work your cardiovascular system, make sure you keep your range of movement by doing the following:

- Always move through the complete range of movement when you perform any of the warm-up moves, for example, lift your arm as high and as far back as it will go then swing it all the way forwards and down and back as far as it will go in the other direction. If you simply work half the range of movement all the time, ligaments and muscle fibres can start to tighten, ultimately restricting your natural range.
- Concentrate throughout your toning exercises and, at the end of each workout, stretch the muscles back to their original length.
- Try to include in any programme a session where you concentrate more on developmental stretching (see page 124), so that you become even *more* flexible over time.

What weight should I use?

To find a weight that works your muscles at a safe but intense level, you need to follow what we call the '10-rep max' rule. Read through the examples to discover how to find your '10-rep max'.

The '10-rep max' test

For this test you need some dumbbells of varying weights or ones to which you can add increasing weights.

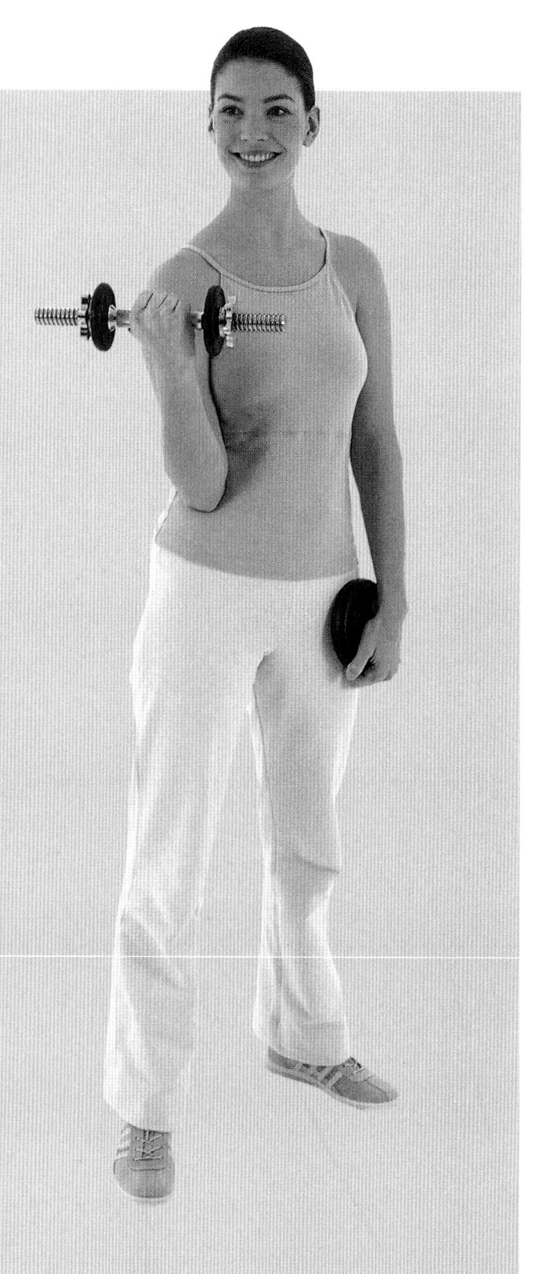

A biceps curl

1 Stand tall with a dumbbell in one hand. Now start to perform a very basic biceps curl, by bending your elbow and lifting the hand towards your shoulder.

2 Hold then release your arm down slowly. Repeat this movement slowly 10 times. Then change sides.

The idea is that on the tenth repetition your muscle should start to 'give up' so that you cannot continue. This is known as 'muscle failure'. If you can work to this failure rate each time, you are working hard enough to see the benefits most quickly.

If after 10 repetitions, however, you feel you could still perform more lifts and your muscle is not crying out for you to stop, then the weight is not heavy enough. Add one small plate to your dumbbell and repeat the testing process again on the other arm.

Once you have found a weight of dumbbell where you are struggling as you perform the tenth repetition then you have found your '10-rep max'.

Go through the same process again, this time performing a triceps extension.

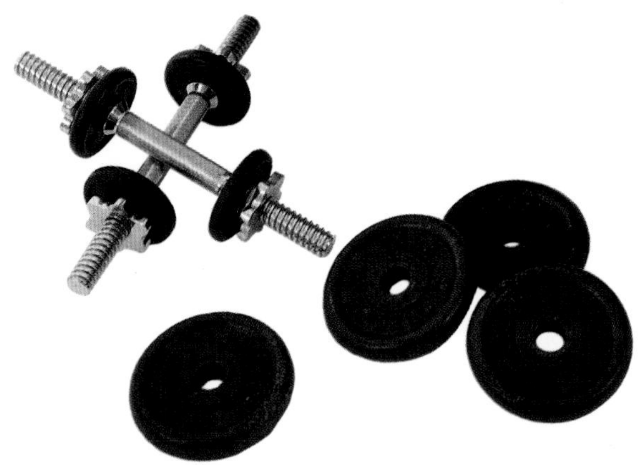

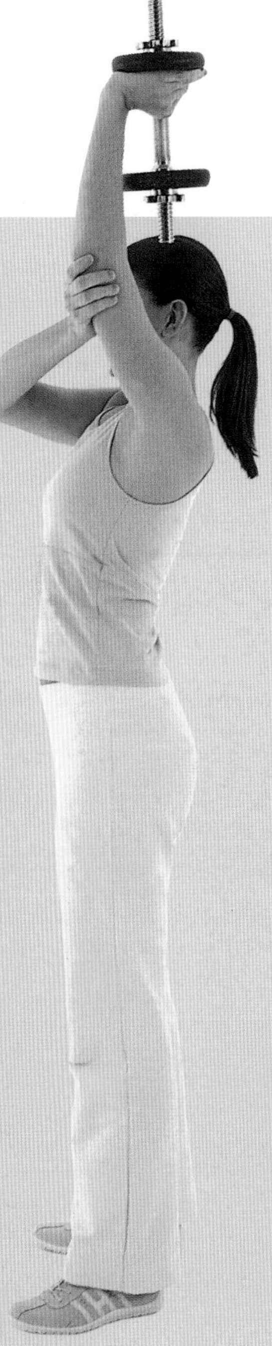

A triceps extension

1 Stand with your feet hip-width apart. Take a dumbbell in one hand and lift your arm towards the ceiling. Then bend your elbow to drop the arm down behind your shoulder. Support your elbow with the other arm, and keep your upper body lifted.

2 Extend the bent arm upwards, pressing the end of the weight towards the ceiling. Keep your abdominals pulled in as you straighten your arm to stop you arching your back. Then lower your arm. Repeat this movement slowly 10 times.

Again, try using different weights until you find your failure rate on repetition ten – you will probably reach failure using a lighter weight for the triceps muscle than for the biceps muscle.

Ideally, you should find your '10-rep max' for each individual exercise as you work through your routine. However, performing the '10-rep max' in these exercises will give you a good indication of the heaviest and lightest weights you might need. Generally you will find that larger muscles such as those in the legs and buttocks will need heavier weights than those in the chest and lower back.

Once you have found your basic '10-rep max', you know you are ready to put in the best possible work in the least amount of repetitions and time.

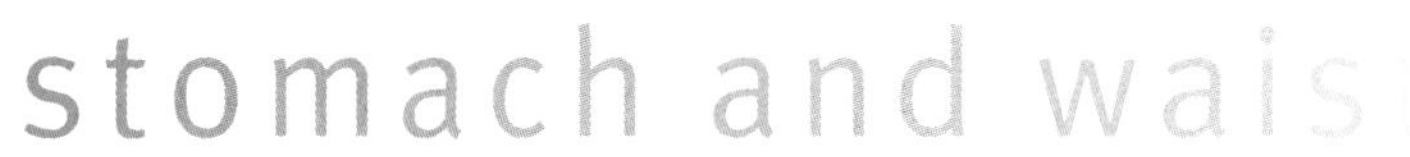

stomach and waist

bottom and hips

legs and thighs

arms and upper body

problem areas

Working with your programme

By now you should have a much better idea of what you are trying to achieve. You may have decided that you need to lose some body fat or simply loosen up, or perhaps that your stomach is your worst area and you need to start work on it immediately.

The body-sculpting programme is divided into four six-week training programmes, each concentrating on sculpting one of four areas of the body. This allows you to focus on your problem areas and make solid gains as you progress from beginners' exercises in Week 1 to the more advanced exercises in Week 6.

The four body areas you can concentrate on are: stomach and waist, bottom and hips, legs and thighs, and upper body and arms. When you have finished a six-week onslaught on one body area you may want to move on to target another area. With the body sculpting programme, you have – if you need it – 24 weeks of constantly challenging and changing workouts.

Each body-sculpting workout comprises a warm-up session, a CV exercise, a balancing exercise, three toning exercises and a stretching-out session, as outlined below.

Warm-up session

This is essential for readying the body for any form of exercise – both psychologically and physically. As you perform simple rhythmical movements you are warming the muscles and the fluid between the joints, you are preparing the mind and alerting the body that physical and mental concentration will be required.

Spend 10–15 minutes running through the warm-up exercises, adding your own skipping, jumping or dancing movements if you feel like it.

The warm-up exercises are illustrated at the beginning of each six-week programme but should be undertaken before every workout.

CV exercise

Improving the performance of your heart and lungs is crucial to feeling fit and full of energy. Such exercise will also help you burn excess body fat. Each week's programme includes a CV exercise that you should try to do after the warm-up. Persevere so that eventually you can keep the exercise going for at least 20 minutes. With practice you can start to add the different CV suggestions together to vary your routine. The important thing is to keep going and build up to 20–30 minutes.

Balancing exercise

Your body-sculpting regime for each week includes a balance exercise. When you balance on one part of your body, the rest of your body has to work harder to realign and hold itself so that it doesn't collapse or you don't topple over. Balancing works the smaller supporting, or postural, muscles and really tightens the whole body. With all the balancing exercises, you need to pull up on your abdominals and keep breathing! With regular balancing work you will notice that you have greater coordination and control over your body.

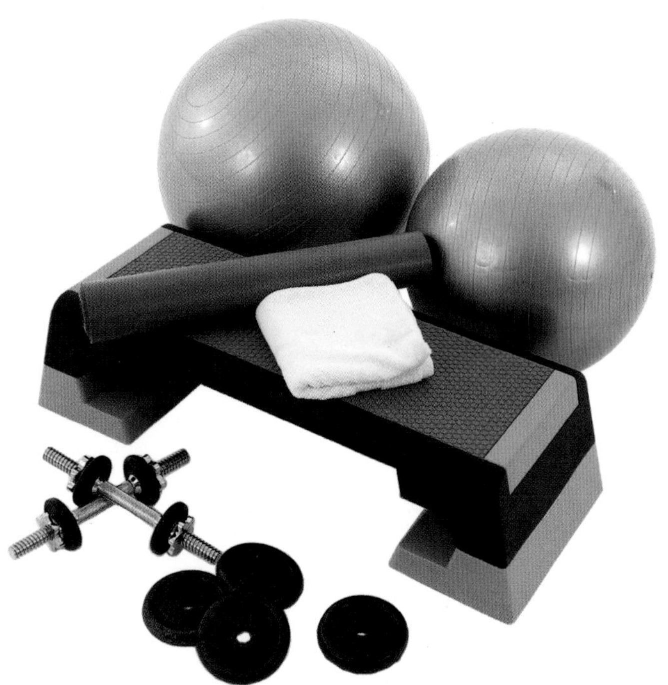

Toning exercises

These comprise the main bulk of your body-sculpting programme and there are three toning exercises within each week's workout. You should aim to do these three or four times per week. Some of the exercises include weights and some use your own body weight. When you are using the weights aim to use the '10-rep max' guide (see page 34) to get the most out of the exercises. When you are using your own body weight you should aim to keep your body as tensed and as solid as you can.

Start all exercises with a posture pick-up:

- Stand squarely on both feet, checking you are not rolling in or out on your feet
- Push the top of your head skywards and drop your shoulders down
- Contract your abdominals slightly and lift your ribcage so that you feel taller
- Check your tailbone is pointing to the floor and b-r-e-a-t-h-e!

Stretching-out session

After your toning work use the stretching-out session as a chance to wind down and calm your mind and body. Stretching and lengthening your muscles helps realign your body after exercise. Repeat the stretching-out session (illustrated at the end of each six-week programme) after each and every workout.

Equipment needed

You will need some equipment for your workouts. Get yourself some good-quality dumbbells that can be altered in weight. They should have solid screw-on locks and a variety of different plates you can add on to the ends to alter the weight for the different exercises (see the '10-rep max' test, page 34).

You will also need a good-quality mat to lie on when stretching and performing toning exercises lying down. Make sure you have a comfortable, draught-free room in which to exercise, it also needs to be free of any ornaments you may knock flying!

Your body-sculpting workout

The following components make up each workout, which should be done three or four times a week for the best results:

- **Warm-ups x 4** (see pages 40, 58, 76 and 94–96)
- **CV work** (building up to 30 minutes)
- **Balance exercise**
- **Toning exercises x 3** (using the relevant week)
- **Stretches x 4** (see pages 54, 72, 90 and 108)

STOMACH AND WAIST

Aim to do the stomach and waist exercise routine three or four times each week for the full six weeks for the best results.

Always precede each session with the warm-up exercises below and finish with the stretches on page 56.

Warm-up exercises

These warm-up movements should be performed before each session of stomach exercises to get the blood flowing. Perform these moves as many times as it takes for you to feel warm and really awake – at least 10 minutes.

Begin by marching on the spot for 5 minutes, bringing your knees up high in front of you and swinging your arms. Move on to the first warm-up exercise, but return to marching for 30–40 seconds between each of the following exercises.

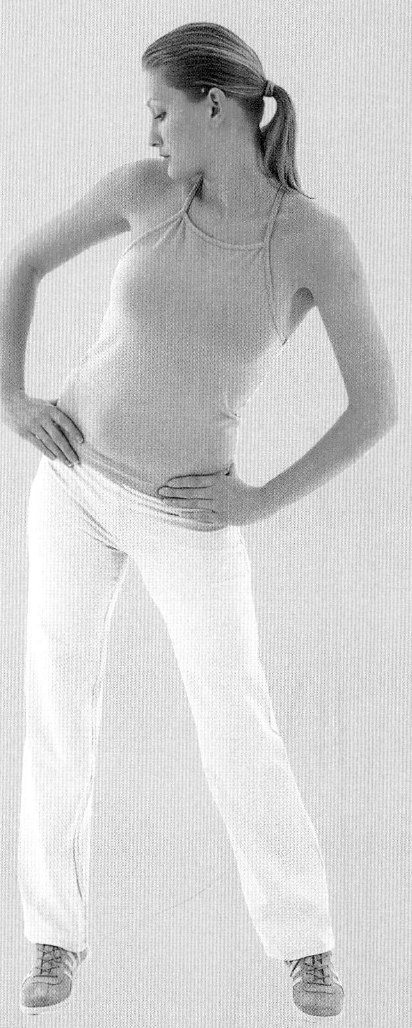

▲1 Hip circles

1 Stand with your feet hip-width apart and your hands on your hips. Start to push your hips out to one side then around in as wide a circle as you can.

2 Circle first one way and then the other. Your upper body should stay fairly straight with your bottom half really moving as you circle your hips. This will warm the torso area and wake up your spine.

2 Waist circles

1 Stand with your hands on your hips as for Hip Circles but this time move your upper body around in a circle, while keeping your lower body fixed.

2 Circle first one way and then the other. Keep going until the move feels smooth and you cannot hear any creaks! This movement will warm up your back and ribs.

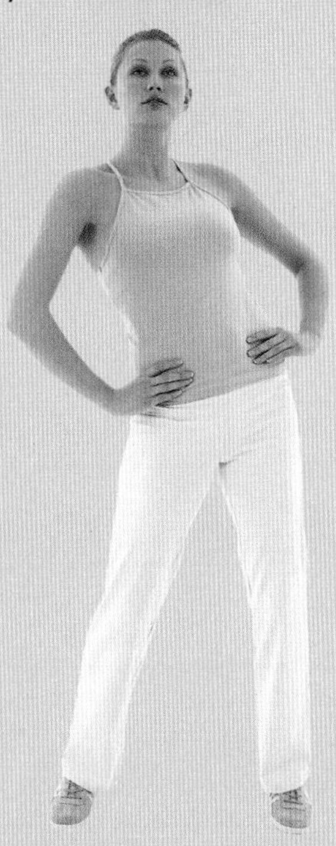

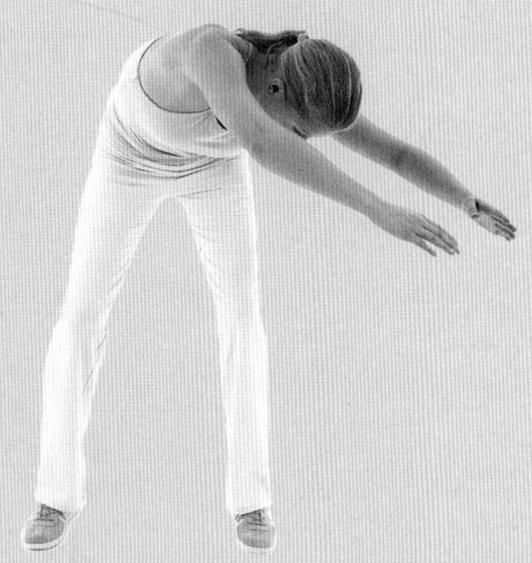

3 Waist circles with straight arms

1 When you have mastered the movement above, try extending your arms. This pulls the body into more of a lean, both forward and backwards, so try the move slowly at first. As you repeat these warm-up moves throughout your six weeks you will find that you can keep the hips fixed and the upper body will really start to move. This builds strength as well as limbering up the torso.

4 Side bends

1 Stand with your feet hip-width apart and your hands on your hips. Lean to one side, letting your head pull sidewards along with your body. Hold this momentarily then lift up and lean to the other side. As with the Waist Circles the hips should be fixed in position.

2 Now extend your arms and see-saw carefully from side to side to warm up the sides of the abdominal muscles (the internal and external obliques).

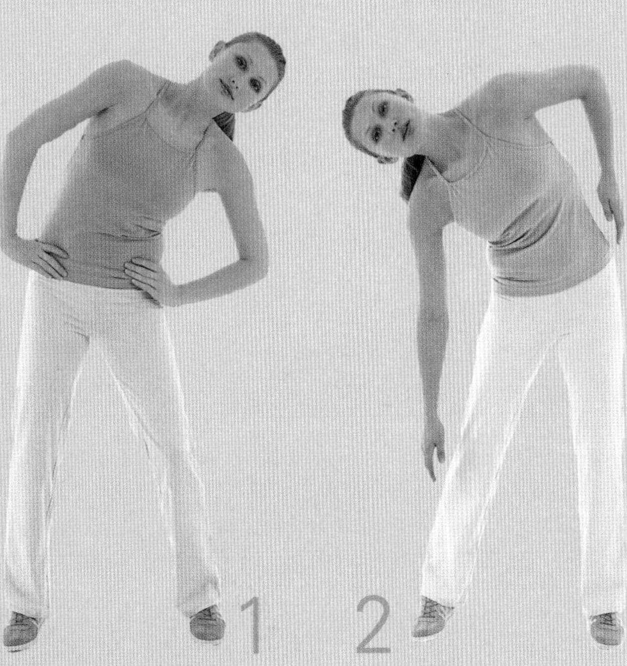

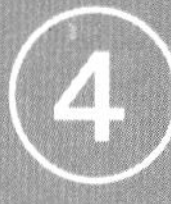

5

6

Stomach and waist | Week 1

▶1 Hop marching

1 March on the spot for 1 minute, as in the warm-up on page 40, but this time lift your legs higher and swing your arms more vigorously.

2 Now as you step down to march push off with the foot so that you are doing a hop on each foot. Continue for 2 minutes.

3 Alternate the march and the hop march and keep going for 15 minutes.

Focus CV

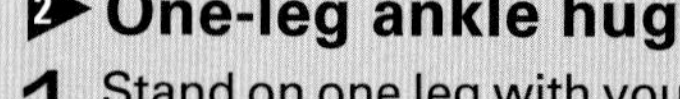

▶2 One-leg ankle hug

1 Stand on one leg with your other foot tucked just next to the ankle. Stand straight and breathe regularly. Hold for 10 breaths in and out. Repeat on the other leg.

Focus Balance

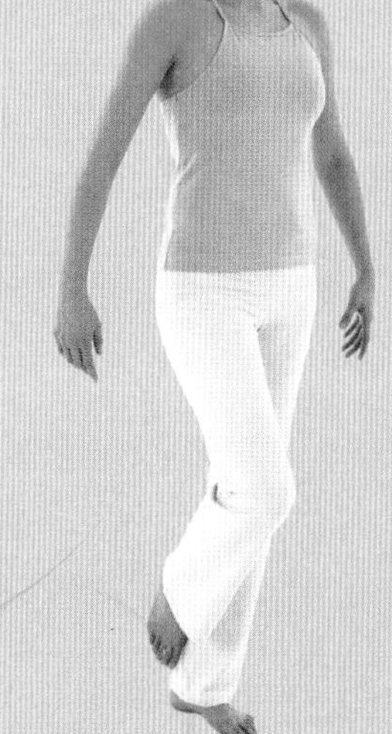

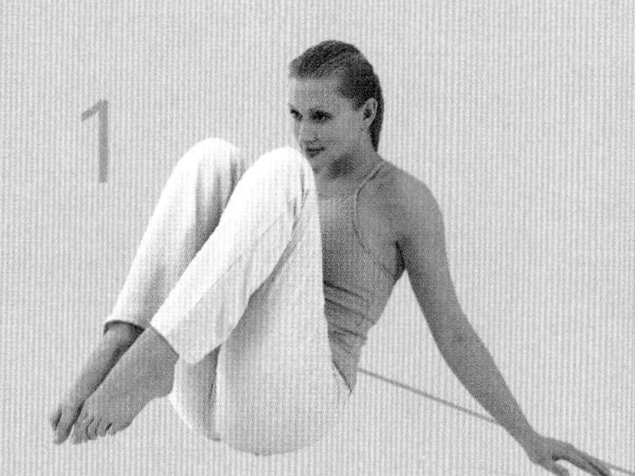

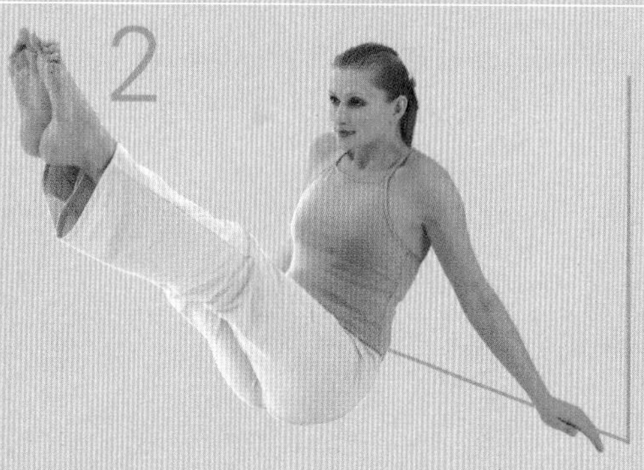

◀3 Hip flexor 1

1 Sit on the floor with your bottom a short distance away from a wall. Lean back to rest your upper back and head against the wall and place your hands down by your sides on the floor for support. Lift and bend both legs into your body.

2 Extend your legs upwards, keeping them pressed together, until they are straight, pulling up on the pelvic floor muscles as you do so. You are now in a V-shape. Hold this position for 5 seconds (or 3 breaths) then bend your legs in again. Don't allow your back to round too much – keep it as straight as you can.

Repeat 20 times
Focus Toning: hip flexors plus inner abdominal muscles which maintain stability

4 Pulse 1

1 Lie on your back with your legs in the air, your knees slightly bent and your hands beneath your head. Lift your upper body off the floor towards your knees as high as you can. Keep your head lifted just off your chest and try to release the weight of your head on to your hands.

2 Now perform 10 small pulsing movements up and down – this is a good way to overload the muscles to make them work harder. Release down to the floor and breathe.

Repeat 4 more times
Focus Toning: front abdominal muscle

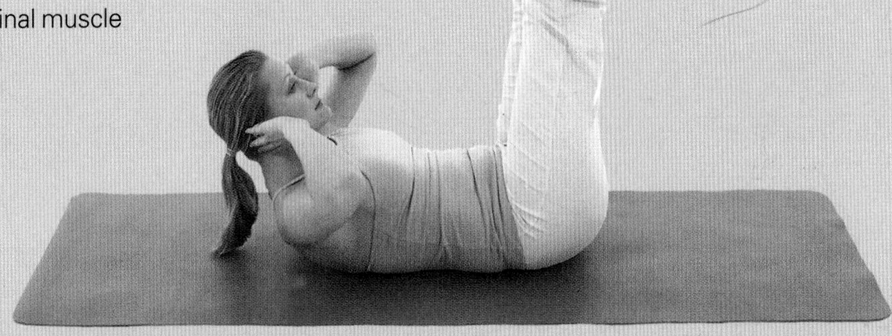

5 Towel curl-up

1 Lie on your back with your knees bent and your feet on the floor. Place a small rolled-up towel beneath your lower back. Place your hands beneath your head then lift your head and shoulders off the floor as high as you can. Hold then release down slowly. The towel allows you to curl up further and really feel the lower part of the rectus abdominal muscle engage.

Repeat 15 times, rest, then repeat another 15 times
Focus Toning: lower part of front abdominal muscle

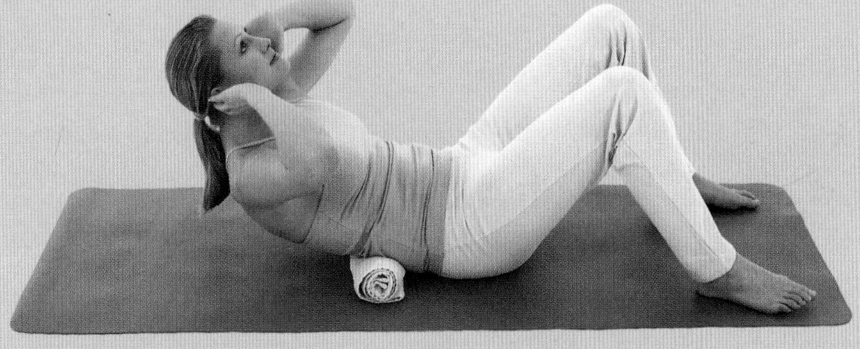

Stomach and waist | Week 2

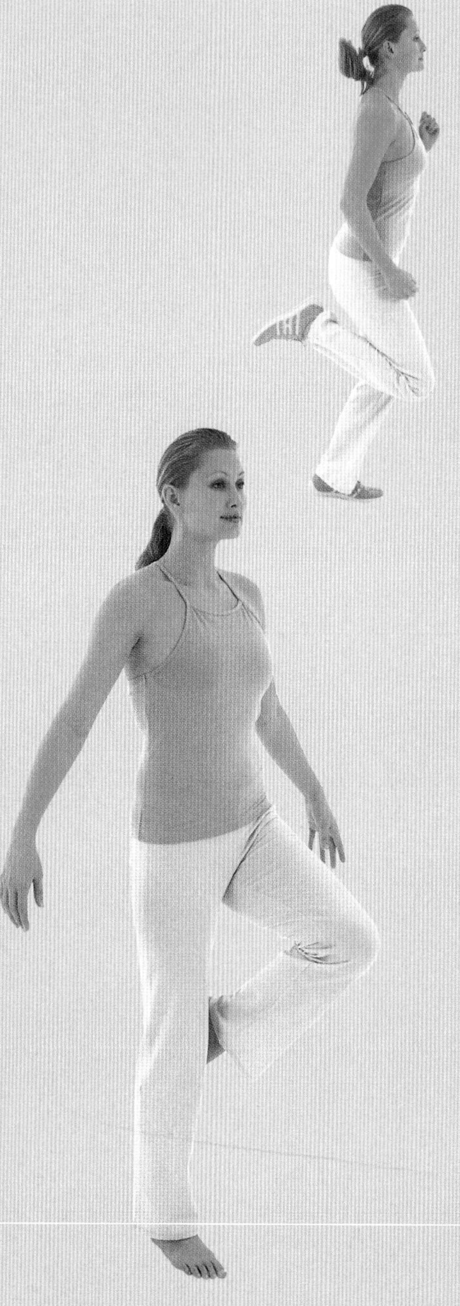

1 Jogging

1 Start with the Hop Marching exercise in Week 1 (see page 42). As you get warmer, increase the marching to a light jog. Put on some fun music and keep jogging. Stay light on your feet and move around the room – and keep going for 15 minutes.

Focus CV

2 One-leg knee hug

1 Stand on one leg. Bring the other foot up until it is level with your knee. Hold your balance in this position for ten breaths. Repeat on the other leg.

Focus Balance

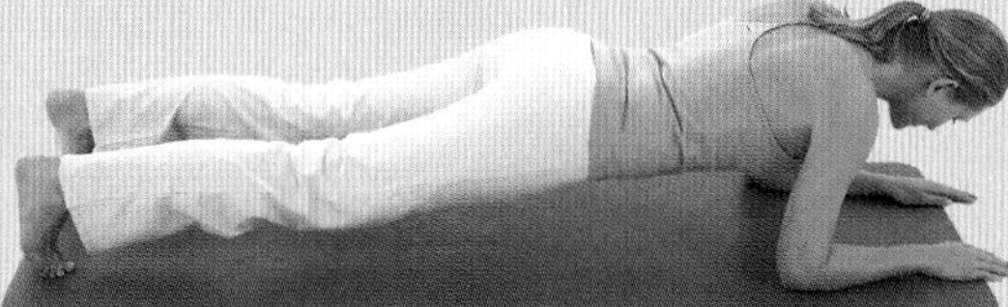

3 Tension hold 1

1 Get down on all fours, resting on your knees and elbows and keeping your back straight. Extend one leg behind you and press your toes into the floor, then do the same with the other foot.

2 You should now be in a solid plank position with your body held rigid, supported only by your feet and elbows. Do not allow the middle of your body to sag but use the abdominal muscles to keep the plank shape. Hold this position for 15 seconds, then rest for 30 seconds.

Repeat 3 more times
Focus Toning: inner abdominal muscle

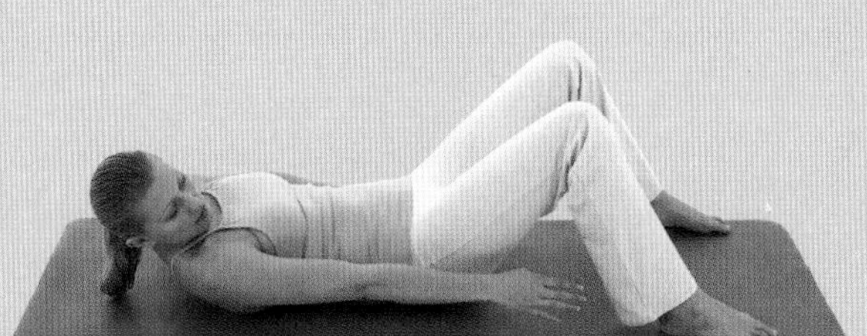

4 Side pulses

1 Lie on your back with your knees bent, your feet pressed firmly into the floor and your arms by your sides. Curl your head and shoulders up off the floor and hold the position, placing your chin where your head feels comfortable.

2 Still lying flat, tilt your body to your right so that your right hand reaches towards your right shin. Perform 20 small pulsing movements towards your shin. Each time contract the oblique muscles at the side of the stomach, then release your body back to the starting position.

Repeat on your left side
Focus Toning: internal and external obliques

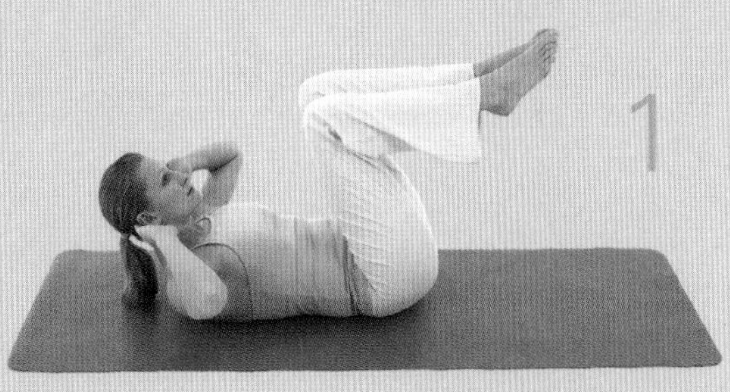

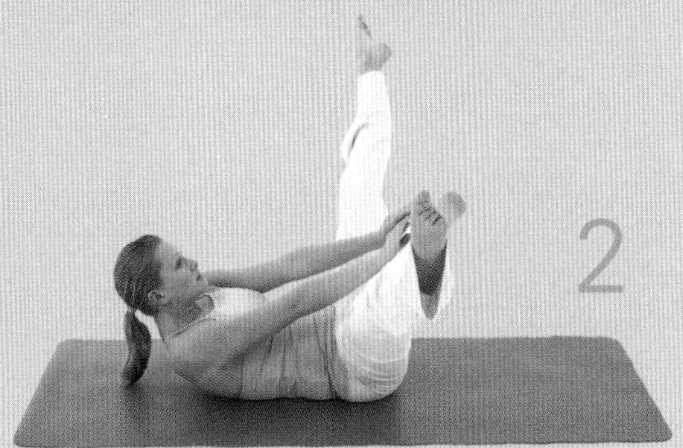

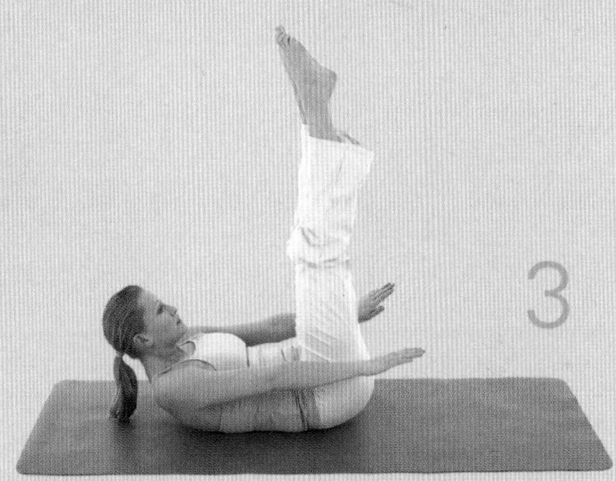

5 Knee pulse routine

1 Lie on your back with your knees pulled in towards your chest and your arms behind your head. Lift your upper body off the floor and perform 20 small pulsing movements towards your knees and back.

2 Now separate your knees into a wide position and do another 20 pulses.

3 Finally, bring the knees together again and perform another 20 pulses. Rest.

Repeat the entire sequence once more
Focus Toning: front abdominal muscle

Stomach and waist | Week 3

▼1 Hopscotch

1 Jump from one foot on to two feet, then back on to one foot, working your way along an imaginary hopscotch board. Keep this going for 20 minutes. If you get too out of breath, just jog on the spot to recover, before carrying on.

Focus CV

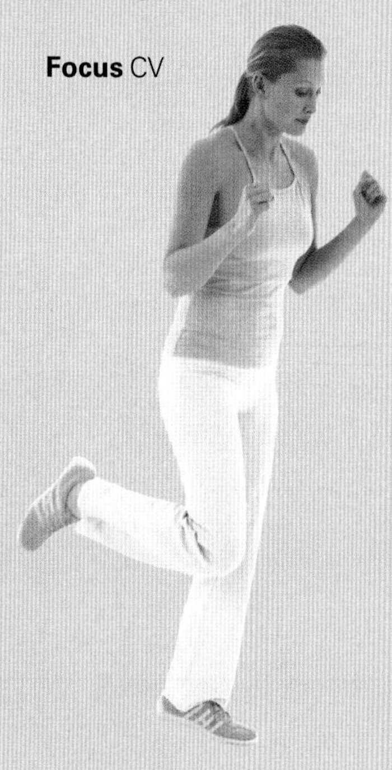

▶2 Straight leg side

1 Stand tall on one leg, extending the other leg out to the side. Keep both legs straight, pulling up in your knees to really straighten them. Extend your arms out to the sides and pull in your abdominals to help you balance. Hold for 10 breaths on each leg.

Focus Balance

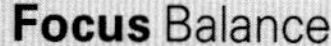

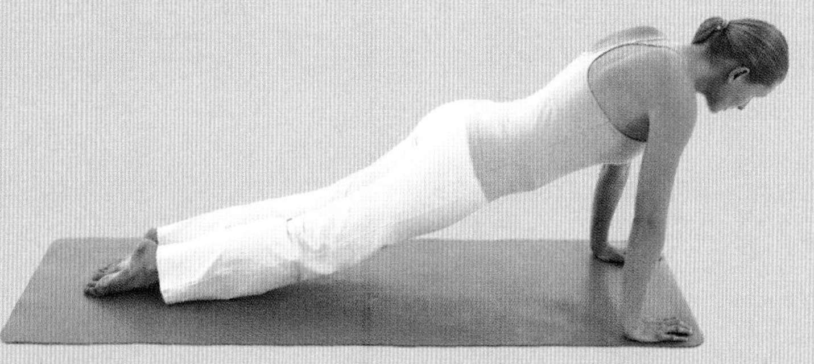

▲3 Tension hold 2

1 Assume a Press-up Position (see page 99) and tuck your feet under so that the tops of your feet are resting on the ground. Hold this position for 15 seconds, making sure you keep your whole body absolutely straight – do not allow your hips to sag towards the floor or your bottom to be pushed up in the air. Hold then rest.

Repeat twice more
Focus Toning: inner abdominal muscle

4 Lower abs 1

1 Lie on your back with your heels against the floor and your hands placed just underneath your hips. Now raise one leg off the ground. Very slowly lower the leg, its heel coming to rest just on the floor, while at the same time raising the other leg off the ground. Straighten your leg as much as you can. Aim to keep your torso pressed towards the ground throughout – don't let the mid-section stick up. Swap the legs over 20 times then rest.

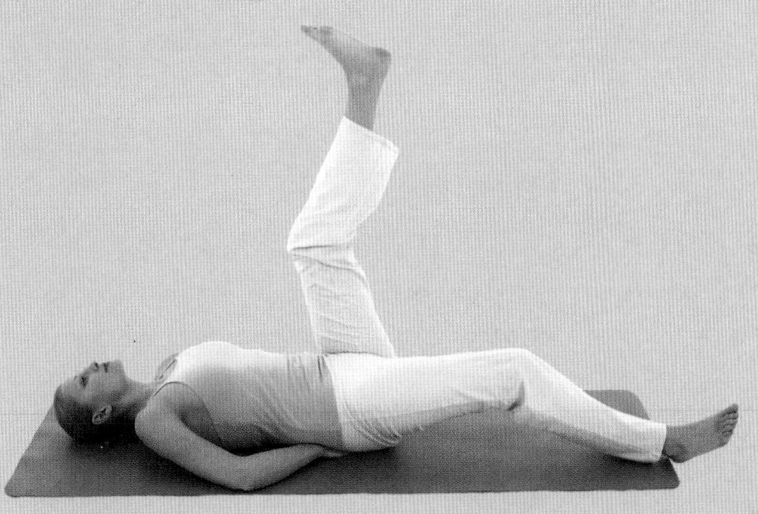

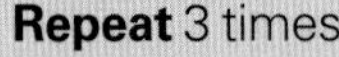

Repeat 3 times
Focus Toning: lower part of front abdominal muscle

5 Hip flexor 2

1 Sit on the floor with your bottom a short distance away from a wall. Lean back to rest your upper back and head against the wall and place your hands down by your sides on the floor for support. Lift and bend both legs into your body. Extend your legs upwards, keeping them pressed together, until they are straight, pulling up on your pelvic floor muscles as you do so. You are now in a V-shape.

2 Now slowly open and close your legs, keeping your back as straight as possible, but using the wall behind to support you.

Repeat 10 open and close movements before slowly lowering your legs to the floor
Focus Toning: hip flexors and inner abdominal muscle

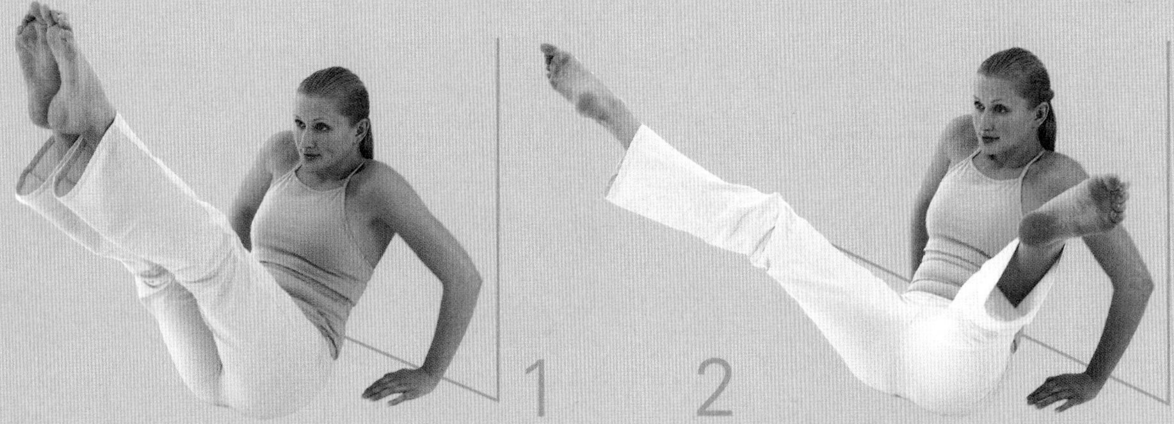

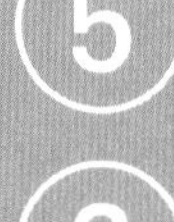

Stomach and waist | Week 4

Grapevines

1 March on the spot then, when you are ready, begin the four-step Grapevine movement, starting from a feet-together position: 1 – step to the side with your left foot; 2 – move your right foot behind you; 3 – step to the side with your left foot again; 4 – bring your right foot to join the left foot.

2 Once you have mastered the move, use it to go to both the left and the right. Intersperse the move with some marching on the spot and the Hop Marching from Week 1 (see page 42). Try to keep this going for at least 10–15 minutes.

Focus CV

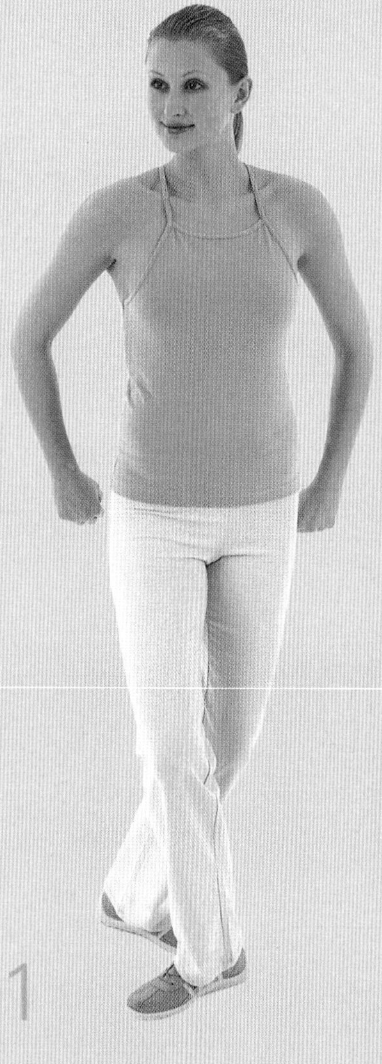

1

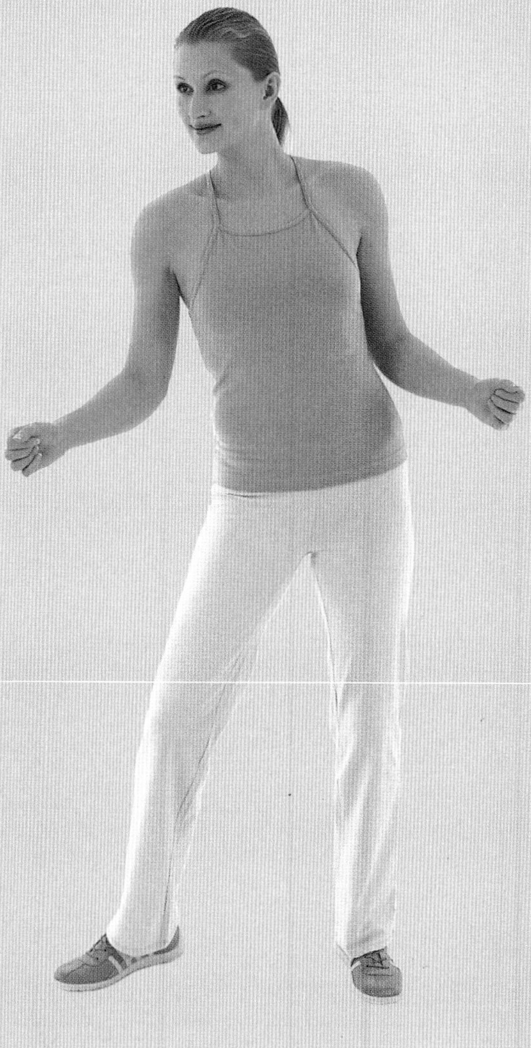

2

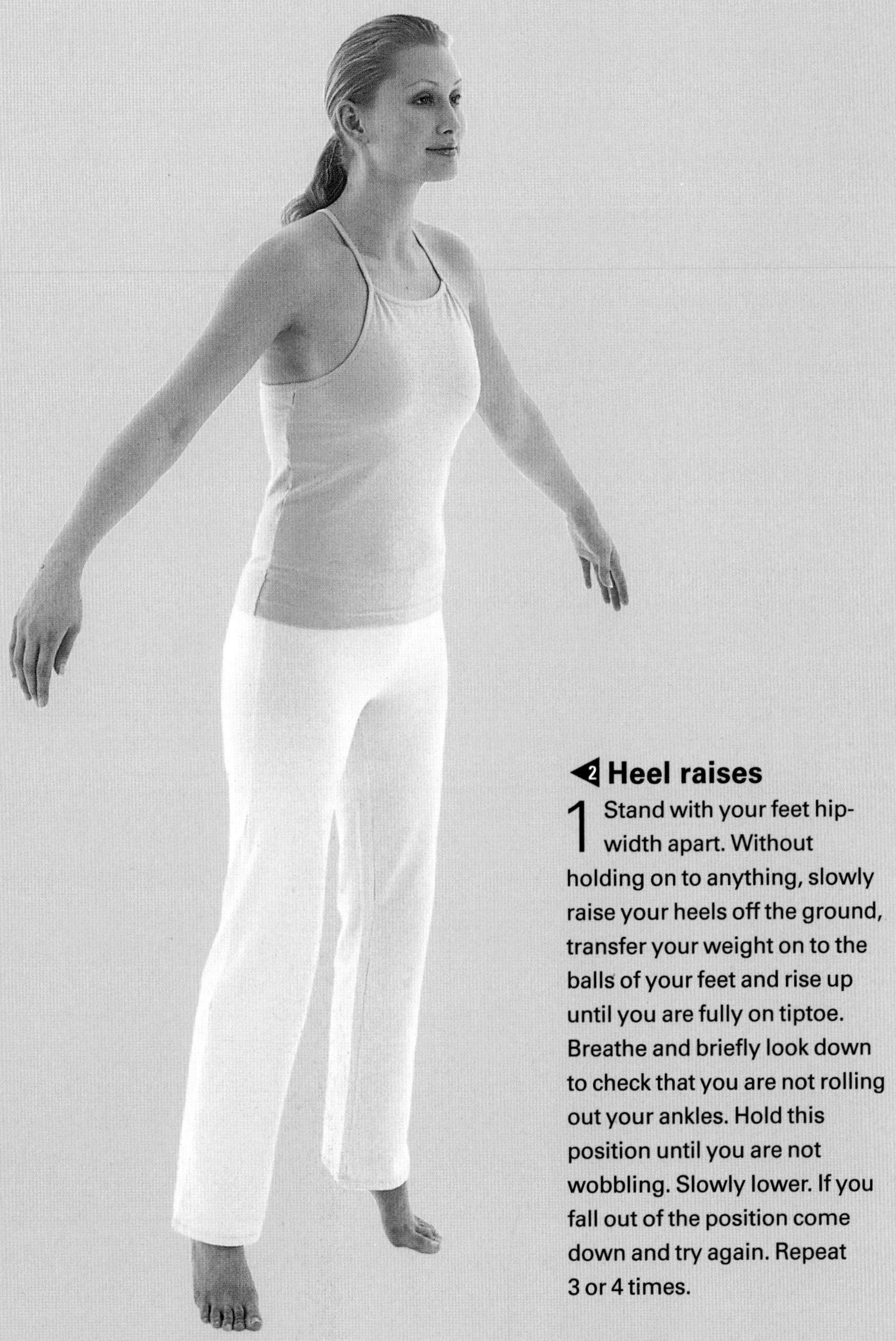

◀2 Heel raises

1 Stand with your feet hip-width apart. Without holding on to anything, slowly raise your heels off the ground, transfer your weight on to the balls of your feet and rise up until you are fully on tiptoe. Breathe and briefly look down to check that you are not rolling out your ankles. Hold this position until you are not wobbling. Slowly lower. If you fall out of the position come down and try again. Repeat 3 or 4 times.

Focus Balance

Stomach and waist

Week 4

3 Yoga arch

1 Get down on all fours, resting on your hands and knees, which should be hip-width apart.

2 Lift your knees off the ground and straighten your legs. At the same time arch your spine and lift your head upwards. You are now in an arched position. Hold this for five breaths then release back on to your knees. Keep the abdominals working to lift your body so it does not sag, but is *held* in position.

Repeat twice more
Focus Toning: spine flexibility and all the abdominals

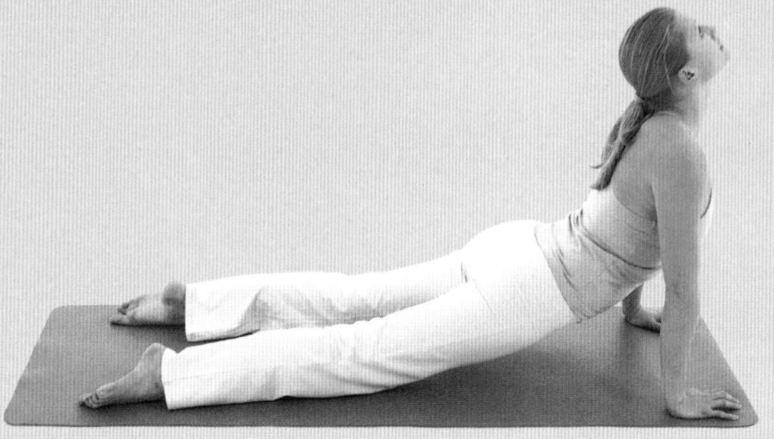

4 Shoot-outs

1 Sit on the floor with your knees bent and your hands flat on the floor behind you to provide support. Your feet should be lifted slightly off the ground.

2 Lean backwards and shoot both legs out in front of you – don't let them touch the floor. Bring your legs back to the starting position. Do 25 shoot-outs. Rest for 30 seconds.

Repeat 25 shoot-outs once more
Focus Toning: all the abdominals, especially the inner abdominal muscle

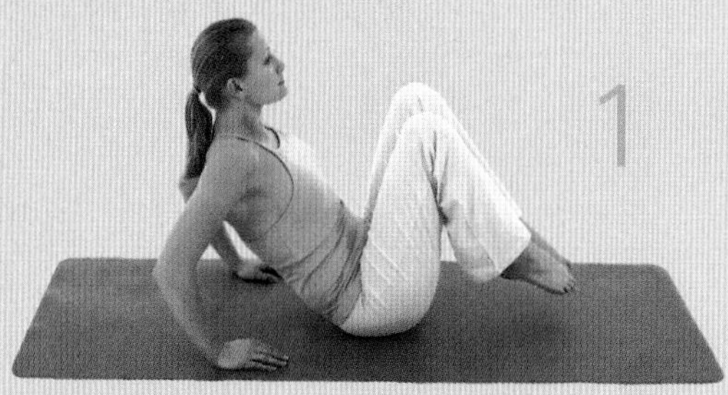
1

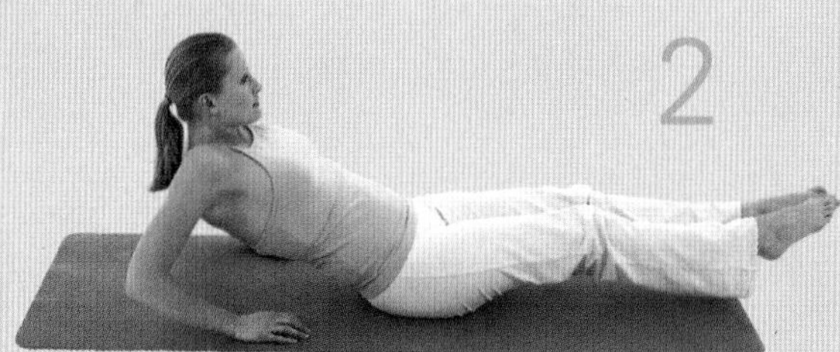
2

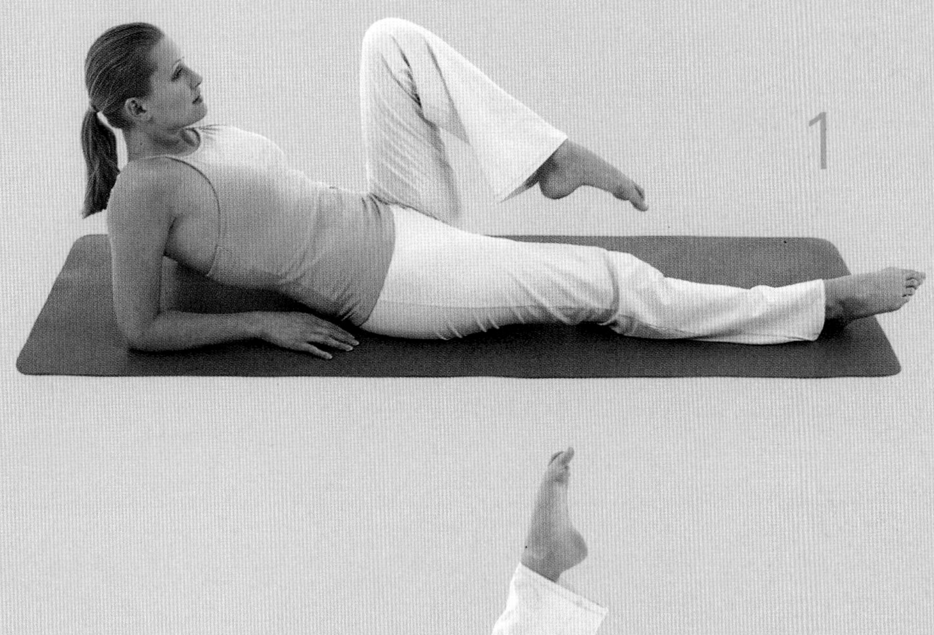

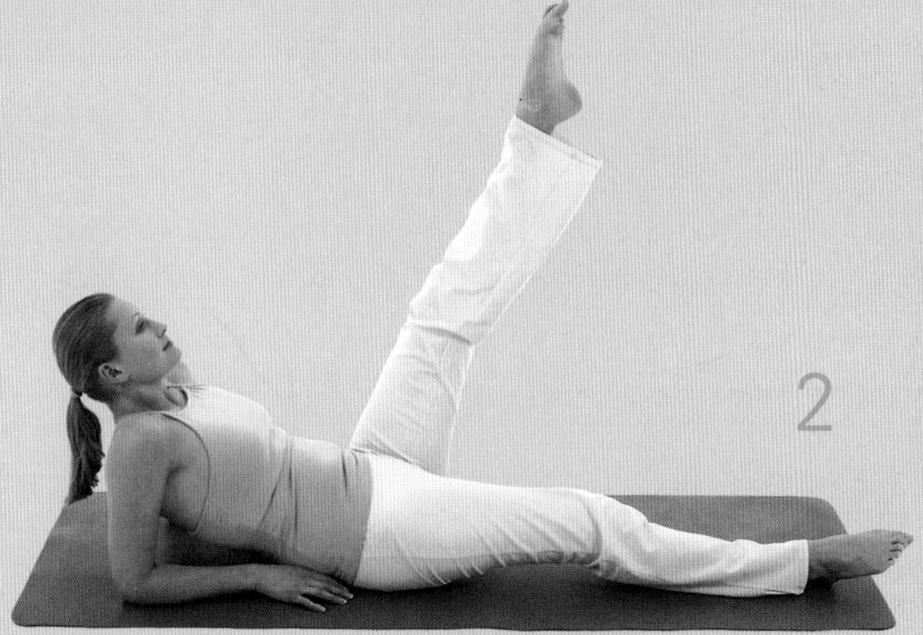

5 One-leg lifts

1 Lie on your back while resting on your elbows behind you. Bend your left leg in towards your chest.

2 Now extend it upwards before slowly lowering it down until it is just resting on the floor. Now bend your right leg in and up in the same manner. Your left leg is still just off the floor. As you lower the right leg, bend the left leg towards your chest again to repeat the cycle.

Repeat 4 times on alternate legs. Rest for 30 seconds, then repeat twice more
Focus Toning: lower part of front abdominal muscle, plus hip flexors

Stomach and waist | Week 5

1 CV combination 1

Make up a routine that lasts 20 minutes by combining all of the following:

- Hop Marching (see page 42)
- Jogging (see page 44)
- Hopscotch (see page 46)
- Grapevines (see page 48)

Keep alternating the four different exercises until you build up a sweat.

Focus CV

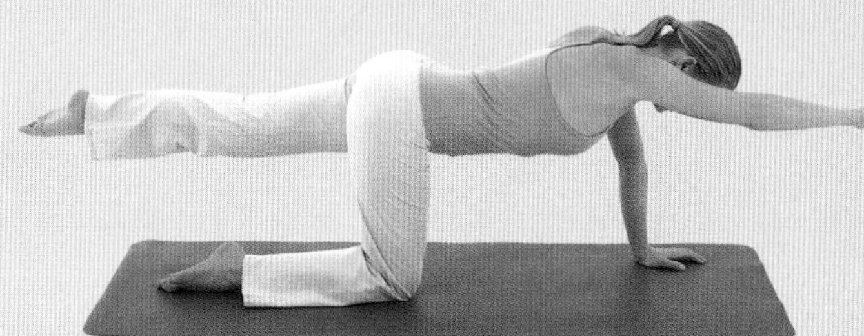

2 All-fours superman 1

1 Get down on all fours, resting on your hands and knees while keeping your back straight. Extend one leg and the opposite arm away from each other and try to balance in this position – sucking in your abdominals for support. Think about sending energy out to the very ends of your fingertips and toes. This will extend your limbs and also help maintain the balance.

2 Do this exercise 3 times with each opposite leg and arm pairing.

Focus Balance

3 Tension hold 3

1 Get down on all fours, resting on your hands and the balls of your feet. As with the All-Fours Superman exercise (right), take one leg and the opposite arm off the floor. Do this gradually as you get used to resting on the remaining limbs. Really extend the energy out beyond the arm and leg to help you maintain the position and remember to breathe. Hold for 8 seconds.

Repeat with the other arm and leg
Focus Toning: inner abdominal muscle

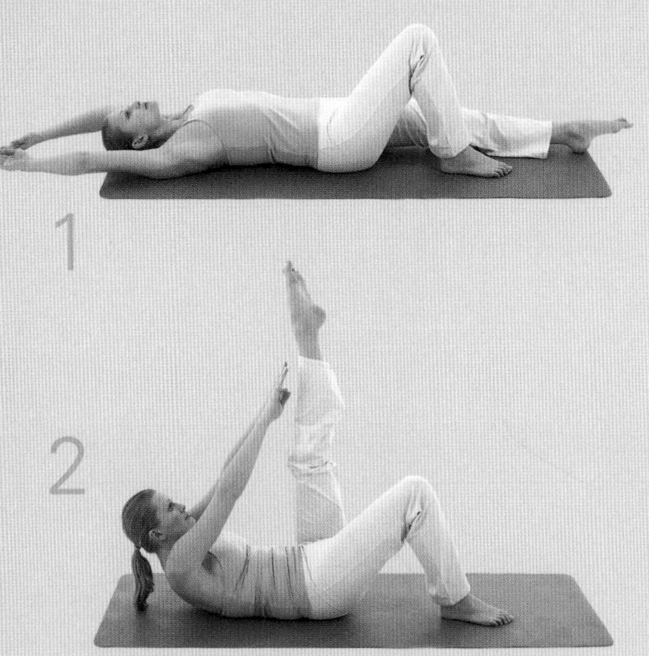

4 One-leg jackknife

1 Lie on your back with your arms extended beyond your head. Bend one leg so that the foot is flat on the floor, and extend the other leg out straight.

2 Now contract your abdominals and lift your arms and the outstretched leg to meet each other. Really contract your mid-section and lift with an impetus to get you right up into an A-shape. This is a tough exercise! Lower your upper body and leg simultaneously.

Repeat 10 times, first with one leg and then the other
Focus Toning: all the abdominal muscles, plus hip flexors

5 Diagonal shoot-outs

1 Sit on the floor with your knees bent and your hands flat on the floor behind you to provide support. Your toes should just brush, but not rest, on the floor.

2 Lean backwards and shoot both legs out to one side – don't let them touch the floor.

3 Bring your legs back to the starting position then shoot them out straight in front of you, then bring them in again and shoot them out to the other side. Shooting out to one side, the centre, then the other side counts as one move.

Repeat the move 15 times. Rest then repeat
Focus Toning: all the abdominal muscles

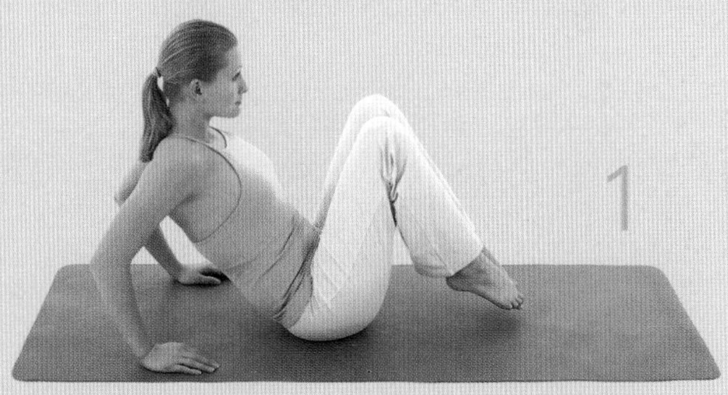

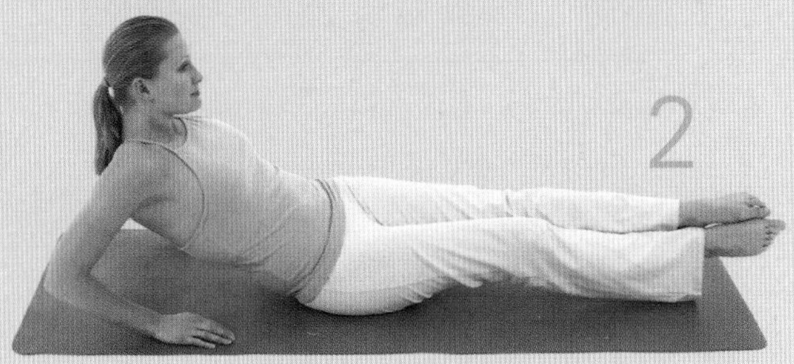

6

Stomach and waist | Week 6

1 CV combination 2

Make up a routine that lasts 30 minutes by combining all of the following:

- Hop Marching (see page 42)
- Jogging (see page 44)
- Hopscotch (see page 46)
- Grapevines (see page 48)

Plus do 15 Star Jumps (see page 82), after each different CV exercise. These tough intervals will push your heart rate up.

Focus CV

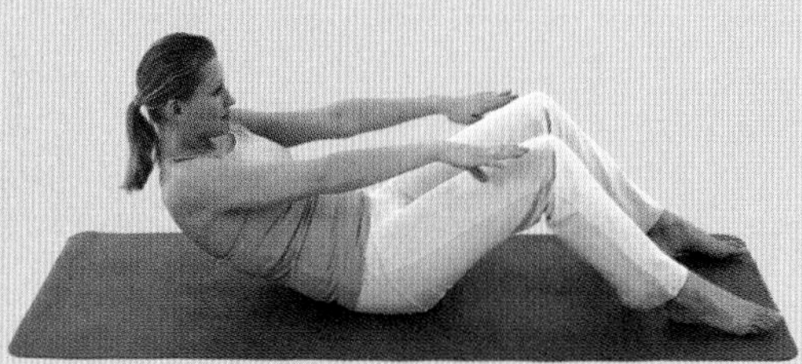

2 Roll-down

1 Sit on the floor with your knees bent, your feet on the floor and your arms straight out in front of you. Slowly lean back and begin to lower yourself to the floor, all the time thinking about pressing each bone of your back (vertebra) towards the floor. Stop halfway down and hold the position for 10 seconds. Use your abdominals to maintain your balance then come back up.

Focus Balance

3 Pulse 2

1 Lie on your back with your legs up in the air and toes pointing to the ceiling and place your hands beneath your head. Perform 10 pulses as in Pulse 1 (see page 43).

2 Now bend one leg, keeping the other leg extended, and pulse for 10. Change over by straightening the bent leg and bending the straight leg and perform 10 more pulses. Finally, extend both legs and do 10 more pulses. Rest.

Repeat Pulse 1 and Pulse 2
Focus Toning: inner and front abdominal muscles

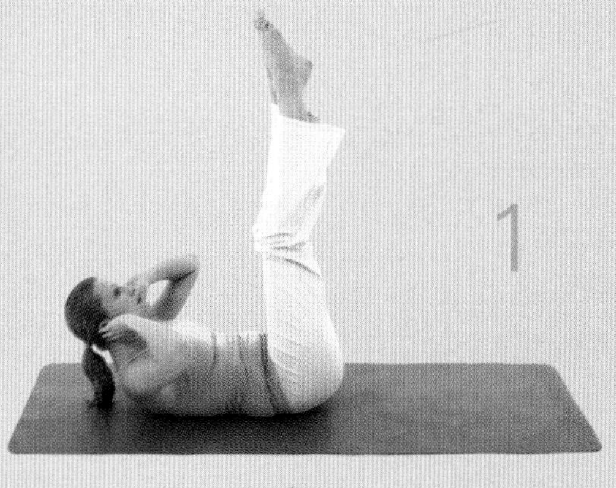
1

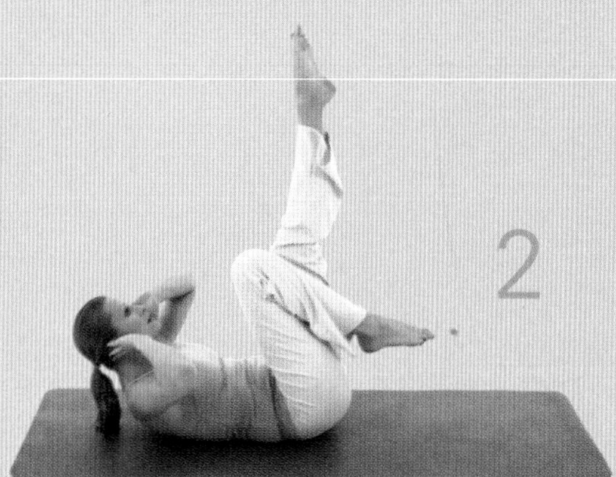
2

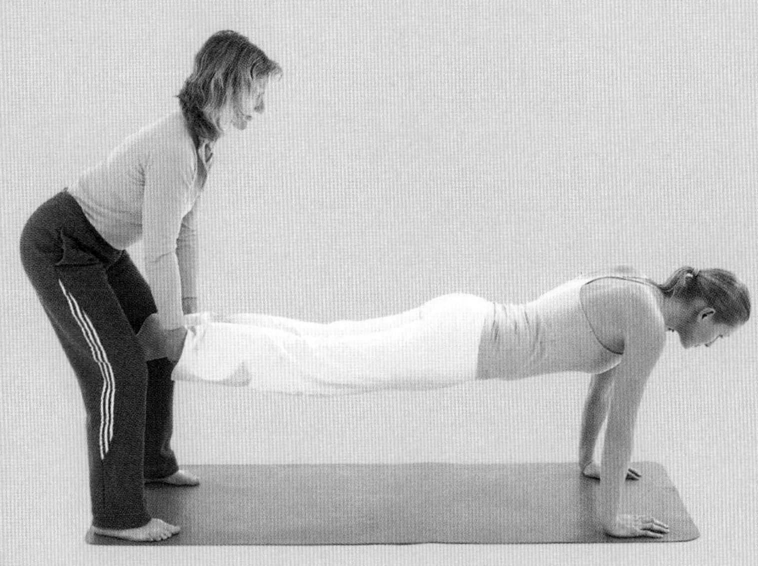

4 Tension hold 4

1 Assume Tension Hold 2 (see page 46) then ask a friend or partner to lift your legs just off the ground and hold for 30 seconds. Whoever is doing the lifting *must* bend their legs in order to take your weight. You should maintain your body tension to such an extent that your partner can tip your lower body up and down as though lifting a plank.

Repeat just twice, with as much rest as you need in between
Focus Toning: inner abdominal muscle

5 Hip flexor 3

1 This is similar to Hip Flexor 2 (see page 47), but without the support of the wall. Sit on the floor with your knees bent and your hands flat on the floor behind you to provide support. Lean backwards, lift and bend both legs into your body. Extend the legs upwards, keeping them pressed together until they are straight – you are now in a V-shape.

2 From this position, open your legs into a wide V-shape and close them again.

Repeat 20 open and close movements before slowly lowering your legs to the floor
Focus Toning: hip flexors, inner abdominal muscle and front thigh muscles

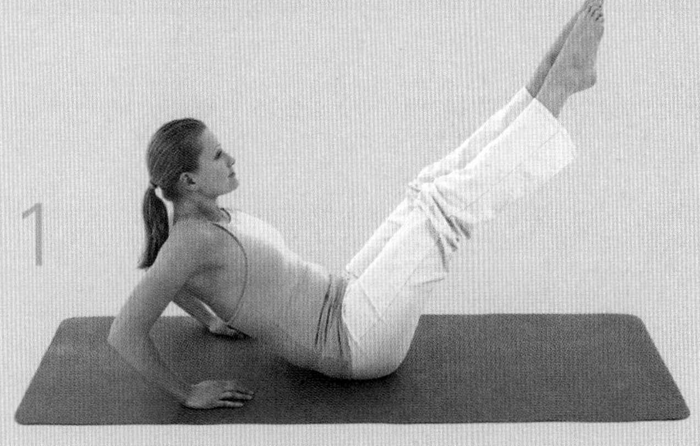
1

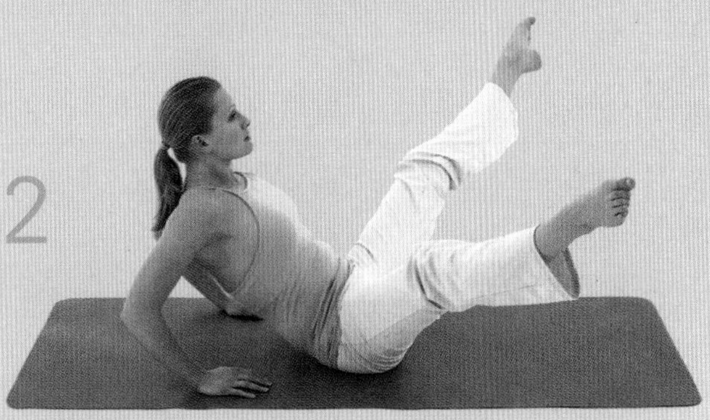
2

STOMACH AND WAIST

1

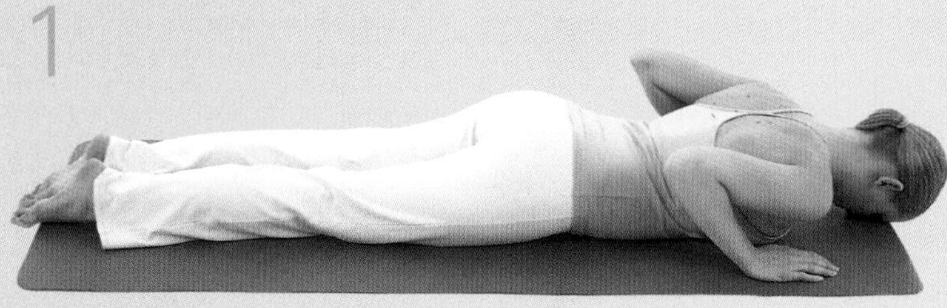

2

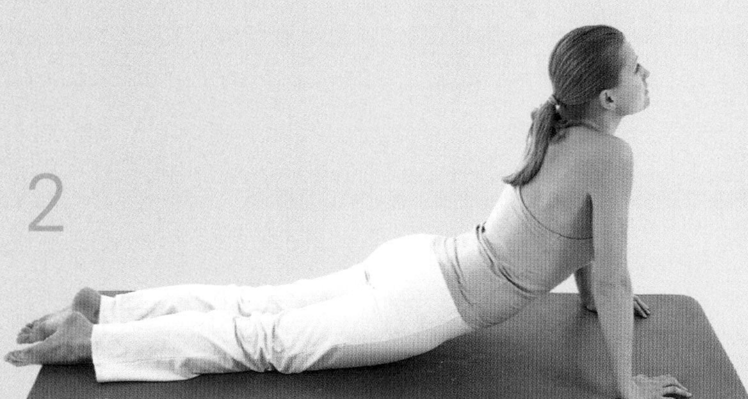

◀1 Cobra stretch

1 Lie on your stomach and place your hands on the floor beneath your shoulders.

2 Gently push with your hands to lift your head and shoulders off the floor, thereby arching your back. Push your hips into the floor to give your abdominals a really good stretch. Hold for 8–10 seconds, release and repeat.

▼2 Lie hug

1 Lie on your back and bring your knees into your chest. Hold your knees for a moment and breathe normally.

2 Now breathe in and as you breathe out pull the knees into your chest a little further. You will feel the stretch across your lower back. Hold this position for 8–10 seconds, then release and repeat.

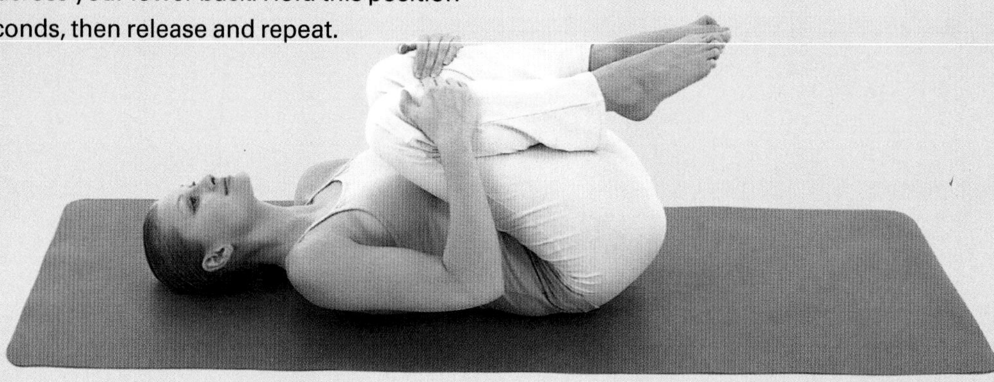

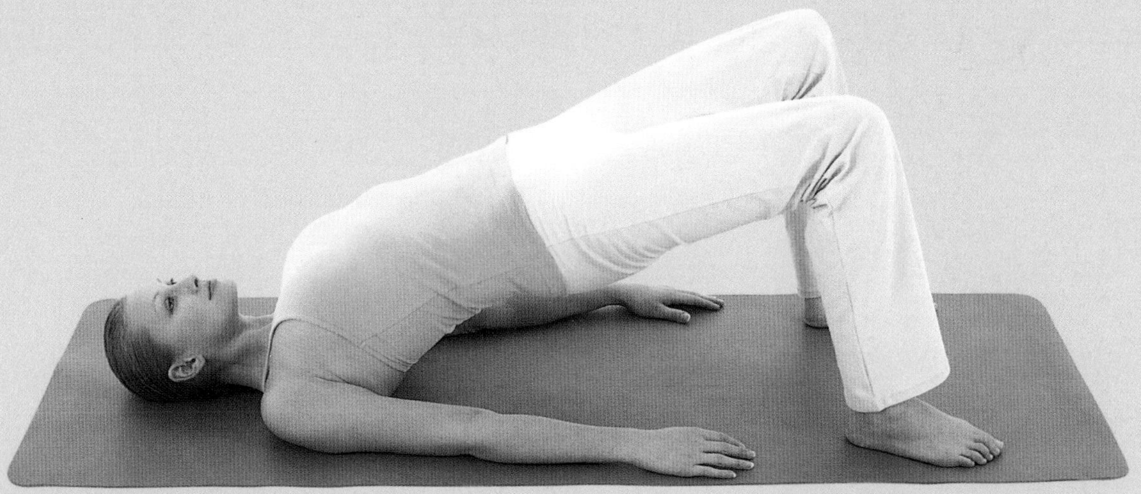

Lie lift

1 Lie on your back with your knees bent and your feet on the floor. Push your hips up into the air and hold the position for 20 seconds. Keep your hips as high as possible and feel the stretch in your abdominals. This position is more like a toning position for the buttocks but it also provides a good stretch for the front of the body.

Reach and lie

1 Lie on your back and extend your arms beyond your head. Press your heels into the floor and stretch out as far as you can at both ends.

2 Then allow your body to relax into the floor for 15 breaths, feeling your muscles slacken.

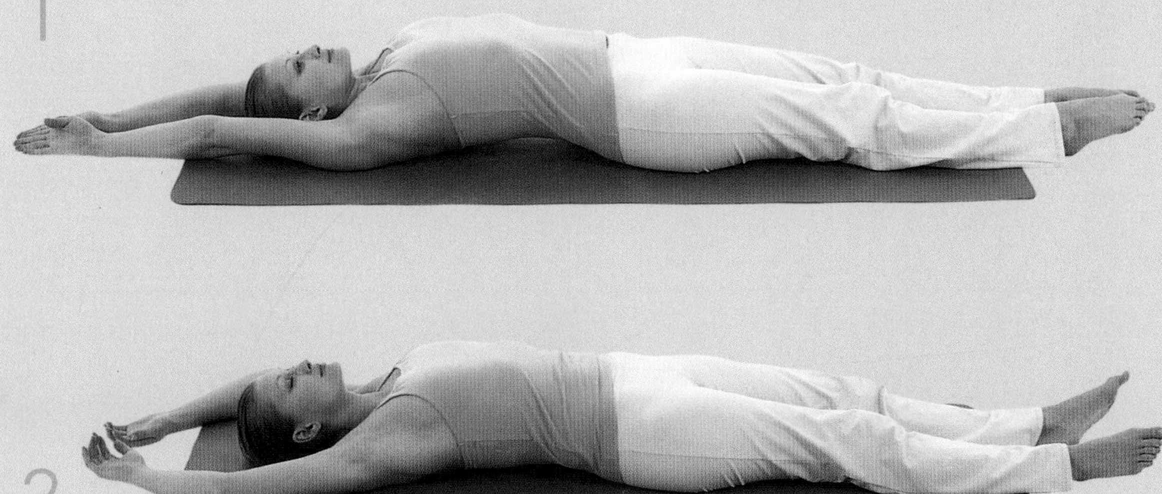

BOTTOM AND HIPS

Aim to do the bottom and hips exercise routine three or four times each week for the full six weeks for the best results.

Always precede each session with the warm-up exercises below and finish with the stretches on page 74.

Warm-up exercises

These warm-up movements should be performed before each session of the bottom and hip exercises to get the blood flowing. Perform these moves as many times as it takes for you to feel warm and really awake – at least 10 minutes.

Begin by marching on the spot for 5 minutes, bringing your knees up high in front of you and swinging your arms. Move on to the first warm-up exercise, but return to marching for 30–40 seconds between each of the following exercises, increasing the pace a little.

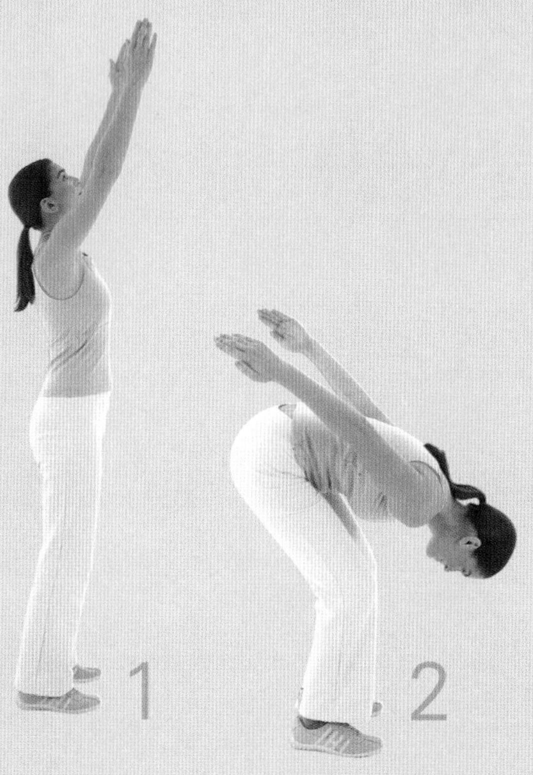

1 Swing downs

1 Stand tall with your arms extended above your head, and with your abdominals and your thigh muscles pulled in.

2 Now swing your arms down past your bent knees, leaning over as you go. As you swing low, straighten your legs briefly then bend them again as you swing back to upright. This exercise will get the blood flowing right down to your head and really warm you as your breathing gets going. Do 8 to 10 good strong swings down and up. If you are feeling energetic as you swing down, add a jump at the bottom of the swing.

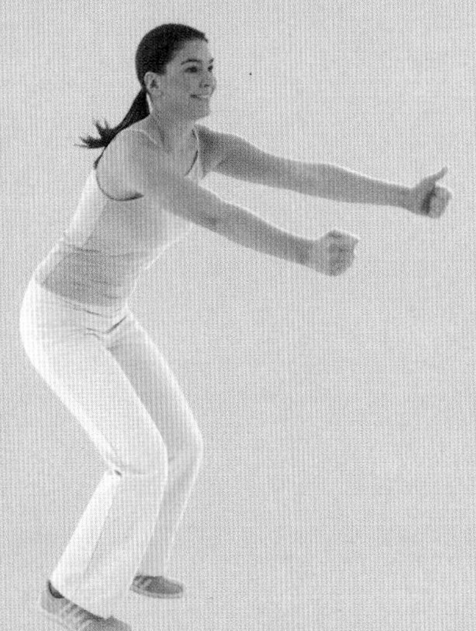

2 Slalom

1 Pretend you are a skier zigzagging down ski runs and jump up in the air landing on both feet. As you land push your hips out to one side as you swing your arms past your body as if skiing. Now jump and land while pushing the hips out to the other side.

2 Do 10 jumps, using your arms to build up some body heat.

3 Forward falls

1 Stand tall then swing one leg out in front of you, stepping into a lunge position. Push off with this foot so that you return to your starting position. Try to hit a point of balance for a few seconds as you push off the foot, just before you bring your feet together.

2 Try these forward falls alternately for 10 repetitions. As you get more confident at these, you can lean your upper body further into the fall.

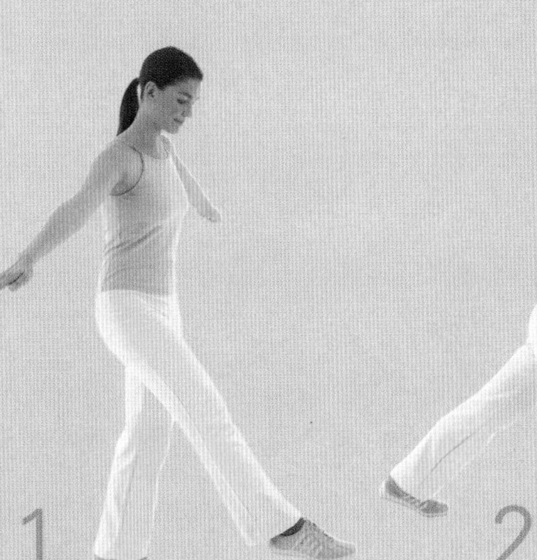

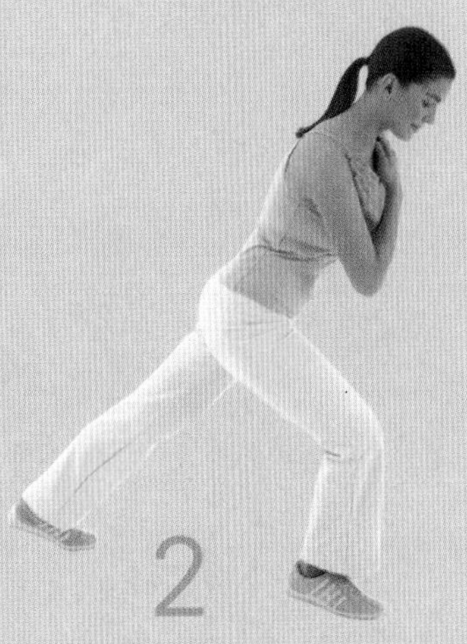

4 Hop sides

1 Stand with your feet together then step to one side, turning your feet out slightly. Lower yourself carefully into a Plié position (see page 61), pressing your legs open as you go down. At the end of the bend, push off the foot to bring your legs together again as you straighten up. Step out to the other side, then push off the other foot in the same way.

2 Once you have mastered this move, add a hop in between. As you push off the outside leg, hop to change legs to the other side. Perform 8 to 10 repetitions of each version of the exercise to get nice and warm for toning your bottom half.

Bottom and hips

Week 1

1 Hop marching

1 March on the spot for 1 minute, as in the warm-up on page 58, but this time lift your legs higher and swing your arms more vigorously.

2 Now as you step down to march push off with the foot so that you are doing a hop on each foot. Continue this for 2 minutes.

3 Alternate the March and the Hop March and keep going for 15 minutes.

Focus CV

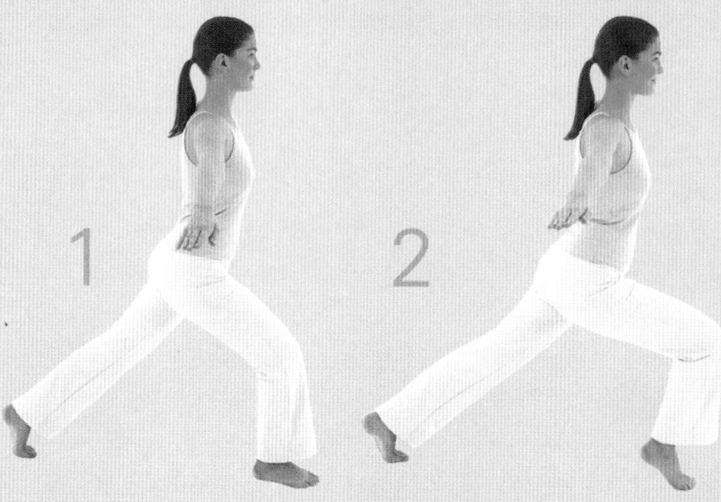

2 Lunge 1

1 Place one leg behind you to assume a lunge position and extend your arms out to the sides. Straighten the back leg, bending the front leg at a right angle. Your back heel will be off the floor. Maintain your balance in this position for several seconds. Feel how the weight of your body is equally placed between both feet as you hold the position.

2 Next, lift the heel of your front foot and try to hold this position briefly. Repeat on the other leg.

Focus Balance

3 Bottom pulse 1

1 Lie on your back with your knees bent and your feet on the floor. Lift your hips off the floor as high as you can. Move your hips, performing 10 small pulsing movements up and down, using the buttock muscles as the impetus of the movement.

2 Pause briefly, then do another 10 pulses, followed by a brief rest and a further 10 pulses. This equates to one set. Rest your hips on the floor and recover.

Repeat the set 4 more times
Focus Toning: buttock muscles

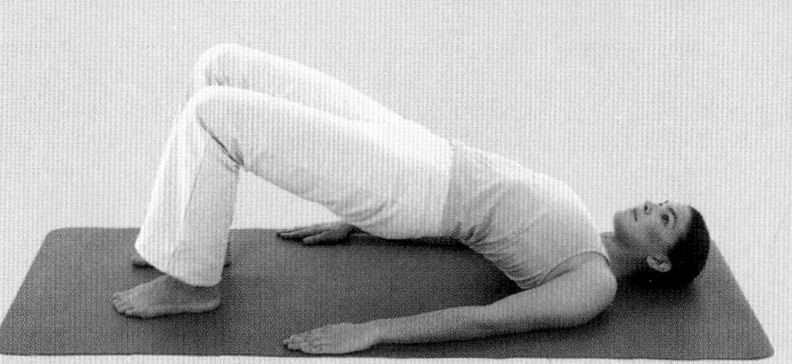

4 Tabletop 1

1 Get down on all fours, resting on your hands and knees and keeping your back straight. Lift one leg out to the side, while keeping the knee bent and your weight equally balanced on the three remaining limbs.

2 Hold this lifted position – you will feel the side of the hip and thigh working – then raise the bent leg slightly higher and then lower again in a pulsing movement. Perform 10 repetitions of the lift on one leg then change to the other side.

Repeat the exercise with 4 sets of 10 repetitions on each side
Focus Toning: hip flexors plus buttock muscles

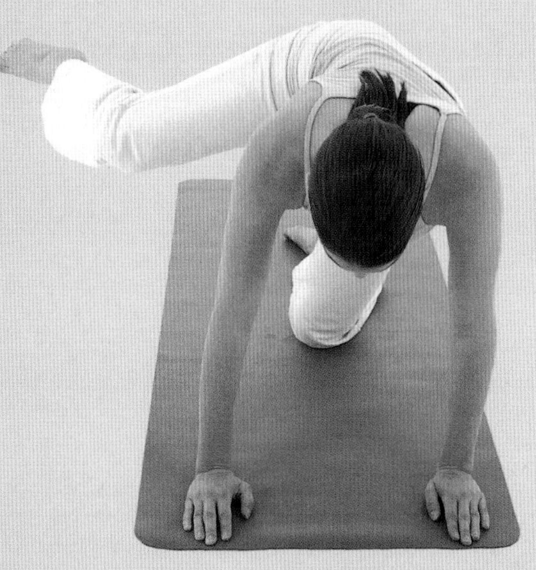

5 Plié 1

1 Stand tall with your feet together and your hands by your sides. Move your weight on to your heels so that you can swivel your toes outwards, using the muscles in the tops of your thighs and in the buttocks to help do the 'turn-out'. Feel as though the turn-out of the knees is happening from the hips downwards, not from the feet upwards.

2 Now slowly begin to bend your knees until you cannot bend them any further without taking your heels off the floor. Keep the turned-out position of your legs as you bend and keep your knees aligned over your toes.

Repeat 5 slow bends and releases back to standing
Focus Toning: hip flexors plus buttock muscles

Bottom and hips | Week 2

◀1 Fake skipping

1 Pretend you have a skipping rope in your hands and jog up and down on the balls of your feet, lifting your feet just off the floor as you swing your forearms downwards.

2 'Skip' forward and backwards and keep going for 15 minutes. This CV exercise should get you really warm!

Focus CV

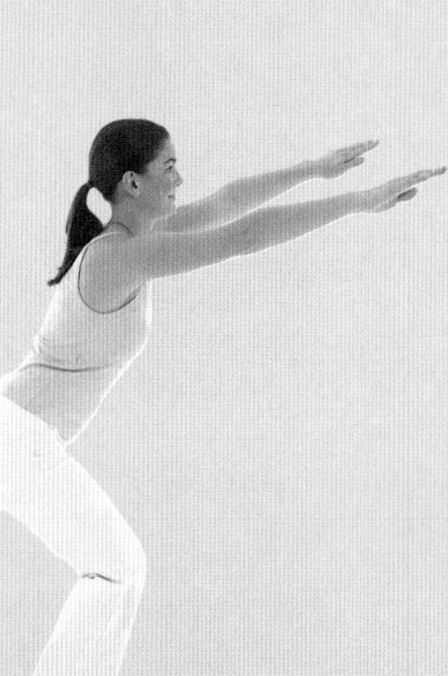

▲2 Lunge 2

1 Assume the Lunge position (see page 60), with your front heel down, and hold your balance.

2 Now push off your back foot and transfer all your weight on to the front foot so that you can tuck the toe of the back foot under. From here, start to slide your back foot away from you as you bend your front knee. Stretch your arms out in front of you as you lower halfway and hold, then slowly raise yourself up again. Repeat on other leg.

Focus Balance

▼3 Hip lift

1 Sit on the floor with your legs outstretched and your hands flat on the floor behind you to provide support. Now lift your hips up into the air and hold the position so that your heels and hands are taking your weight.

2 Contract your buttock muscles to keep your hips lifted as high as possible. Keep breathing and start to drop your hips just a little, then squeeze your buttocks to lift your hips up again.

Repeat pulses 10 times then lower and rest. Repeat the lift and hold, then do a further 10 pulses

Focus Toning: buttock muscles

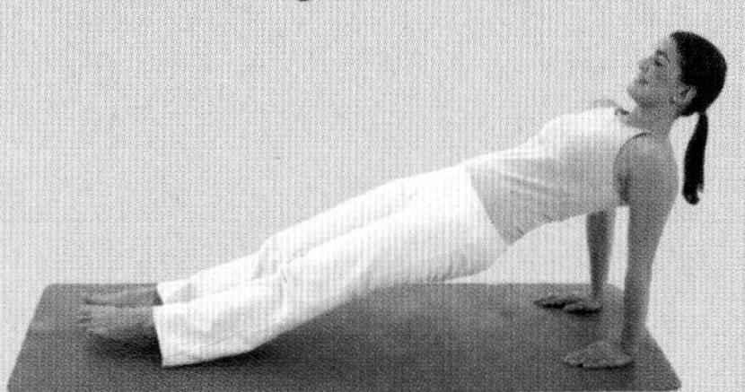

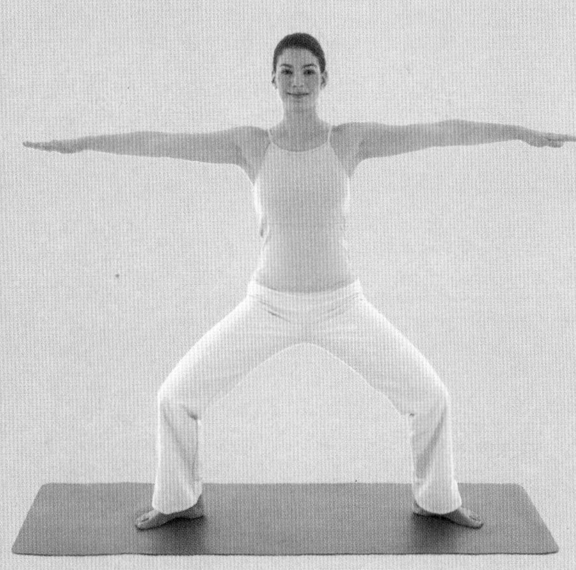

4 Plié 2

1 Stand tall with your legs apart. Turn them out slightly, making sure you do the turn-out from the top of your legs, not just in your feet.

2 Lift your arms out to the sides and slowly begin to bend your knees, pressing them out over your toes. Bend your knees and push your bottom as low as you can without allowing your back to curve, keeping your heels on the ground. Slowly straighten in the same controlled way.

Repeat the Pliés 8 times, shake out your legs, then do another 8

Focus Toning: all buttock muscles, plus hip flexors

5 All-fours contraction

1 Get down on all fours, resting on your hands and knees and keeping your back straight. Lift one knee off the floor and, contracting your stomach and back muscles, try to bring it as near to your nose as possible.

2 From this position push your leg back and up behind you, in a smooth motion, focusing on contracting the buttock muscle.

Repeat these pull-ins and push-outs 10 times on each leg

Focus Toning: buttock muscles

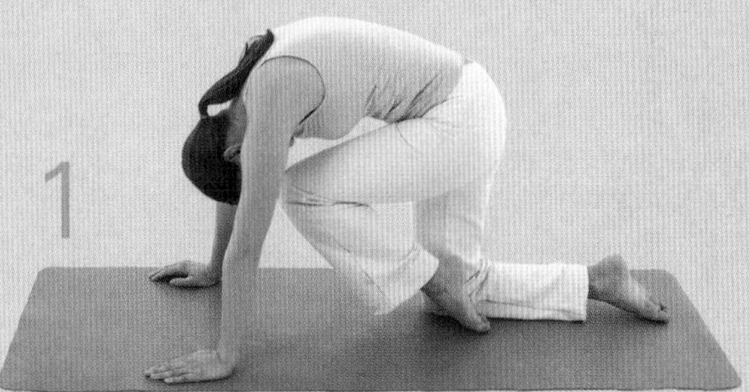

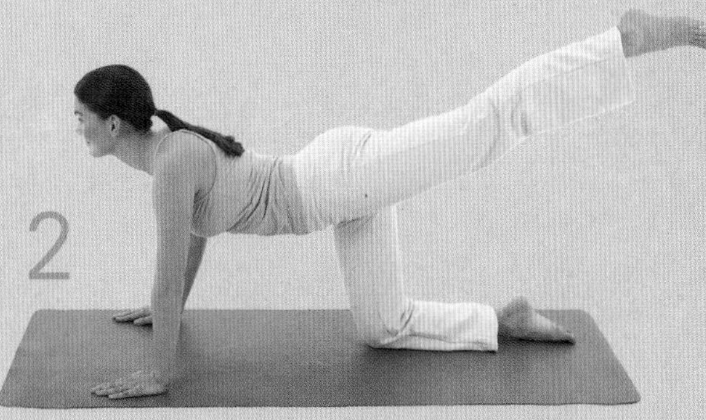

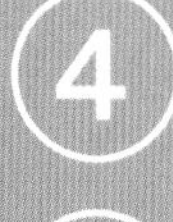
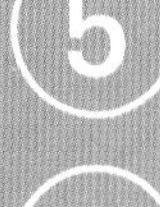

Bottom and hips

Week 3

1 V-dodges

1 Stand with your feet wide apart and your hands on your hips. Bend deeply then, as you lift, come up to one side so that the furthest foot is only just touching the floor. Bend again in the centre and push up to the other side. Do this from side to side working in a smooth rhythm.

2 When you are comfortable with this move, try swinging your arms from side to side as you bend and come up. Keep these combinations going for 15 minutes.

Focus CV

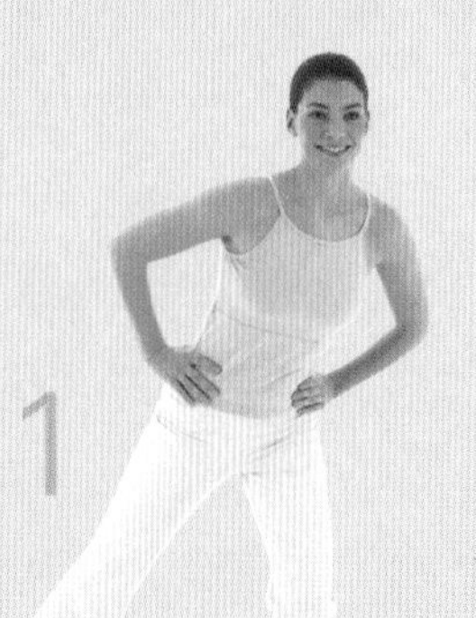

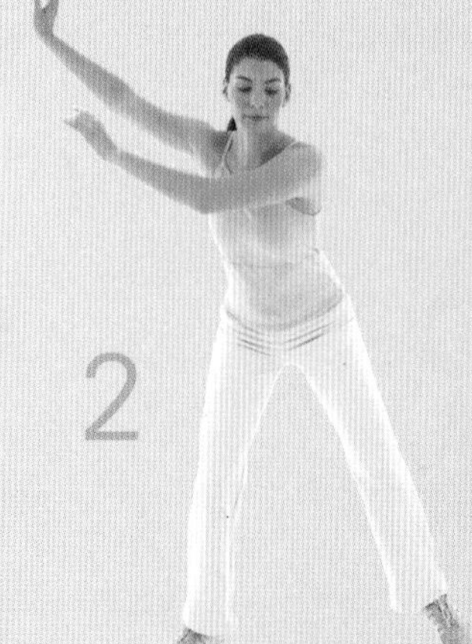

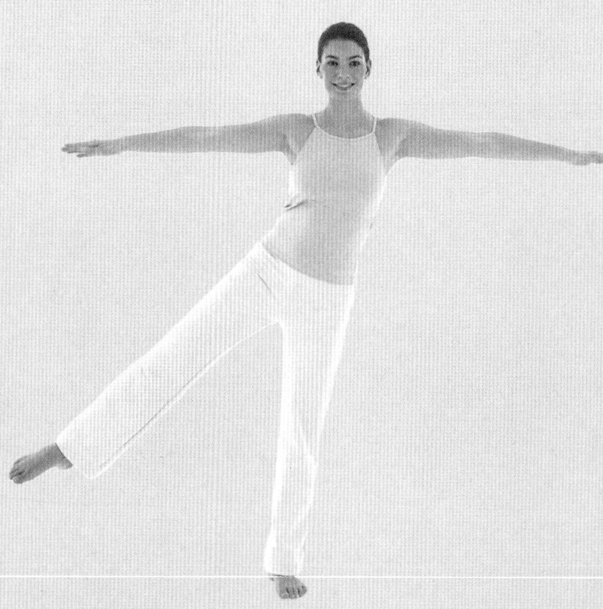

2 Straight leg side

1 Stand tall on one leg, extending the other leg out to the side. Keep both legs straight, pulling up in your knees to really straighten them. Extend your arms out to the sides and pull in on your abdominals to help you balance. Hold for 10 breaths on each leg.

Focus Balance

3 Bottom pulse 2

1 Lie on your back and perform one set of pulses from Bottom Pulse 1 (see page 60).

2 With your hips off the ground, lift one leg in the air and press your hands on to the floor. Now pulse the one leg high up into the air for a count of 10. You will really feel the one buttock working as all the effort is focused on one leg.

Repeat a set of Bottom Pulse 1, then work the other leg. Rest and repeat the whole exercise

Focus Toning: buttock muscles

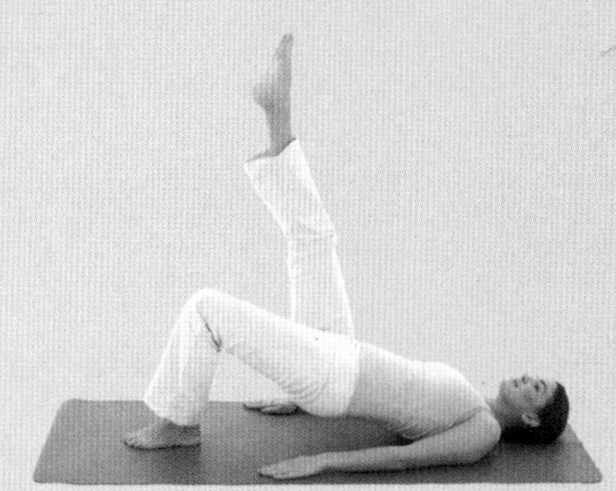

4 Tabletop 2

1 As for Tabletop 1 (see page 61), get down on all fours and lift one bent leg out to the side so that the side of the thigh is parallel with the floor.

2 From this position extend the leg slightly so that it is straighter. Now imagine someone is holding a ball in front of your foot and that you have to circle your foot around it. Perform 8 small circles with your leg, first one way and then the other. Do the same on the other leg.

Repeat 4 times on each leg
Focus Toning: hip flexors plus buttock muscles

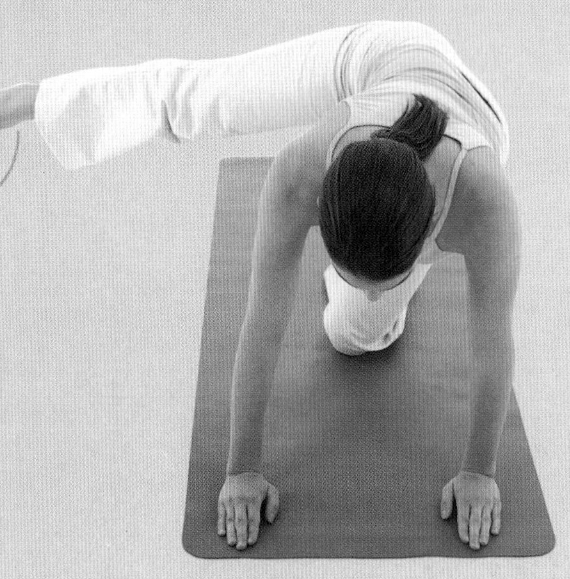

5 Arabesque burner

1 From a standing position lean forwards and place both hands on a chair seat. Suck in your abdominals for support then extend one leg behind you, pointing the foot and lifting the leg as high as you can in the air.

2 Slowly lower the leg back down again. Keep the supporting leg straight by pulling up in your knee and keep both hip bones pointing towards the chair so that you don't twist.

Repeat the lifts 10 times with each leg
Focus Toning: buttock muscles

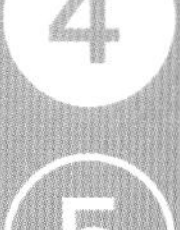

Bottom and hips

Week 4

1 Boxers' jogging

1 Start by marching on the spot to warm up then pick up the pace. Jog on your toes then start to strike your heels lightly on the ground in front of you. Keep your hands up as though you are ready to spar. Move forwards and backwards and 'box' around the room. Keep going for 15 minutes.

Focus CV

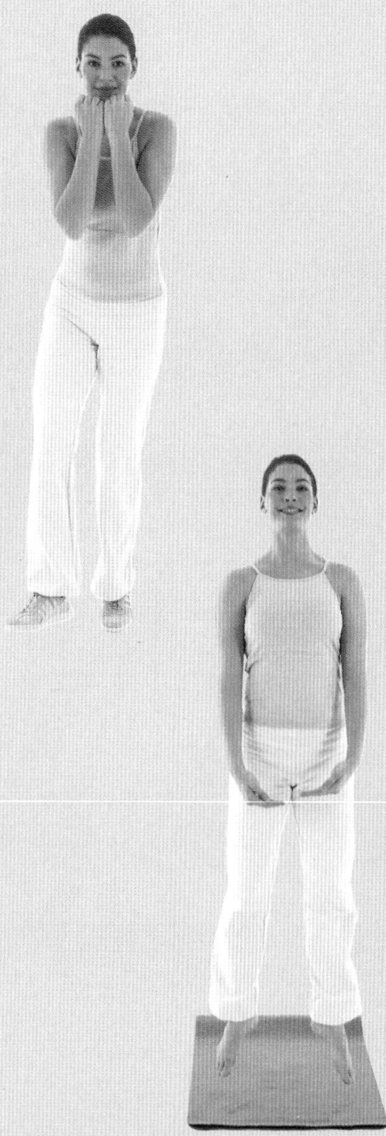

2 Low arabesque

1 Stand tall and lift one leg off the ground. Extend the leg out behind you, tilting your body forwards to counterbalance the leg and stretch your arms out in front of you. Suck in your abdominal muscles to give your body support and help maintain your balance. Try to stretch one end of your body away from the other.

2 Hold this position for 5 breaths then do the same on the other leg.

Focus Balance

3 Little jumps

1 Stand tall and bend your knees to prepare for jumping. Now do 8 small jumps just off the floor. It is important that you land correctly to protect your body, so make sure that your toes strike the floor first when you land and then roll through the balls of your feet to your heels, with your knees bent. This will ensure you absorb the impact of the jump and generate the spring required to perform the next one. Shake out your legs and take a breather before repeating the exercise.

Repeat the exercise with 3 sets of 8 jumps, resting between each set

Focus Toning: hip flexors plus buttock muscles

4 Tabletop 3

1 As for Tabletop 2 (see page 65), get down on all fours and extend one leg out behind you. Keeping your abdominals pulled in, lift your leg up and down 5 times, touching your toes lightly to the floor then lifting the leg up into the air without letting your back arch.

2 Swing your leg around to the side, keeping it straight and perform 5 lifts. Keep your abdominals contracted to avoid arching your back.

Repeat on the other leg
Focus Toning: hip flexors plus buttock muscles

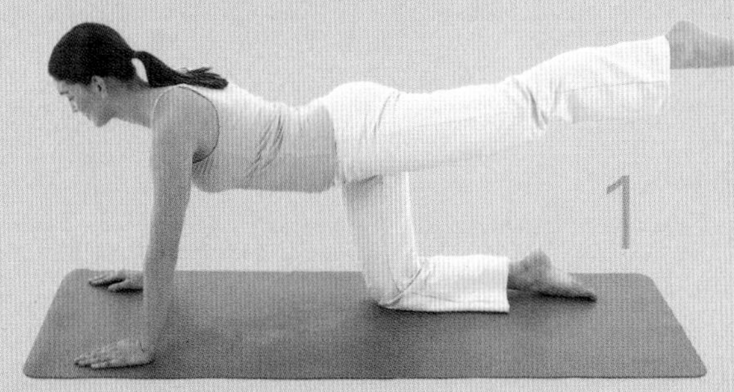

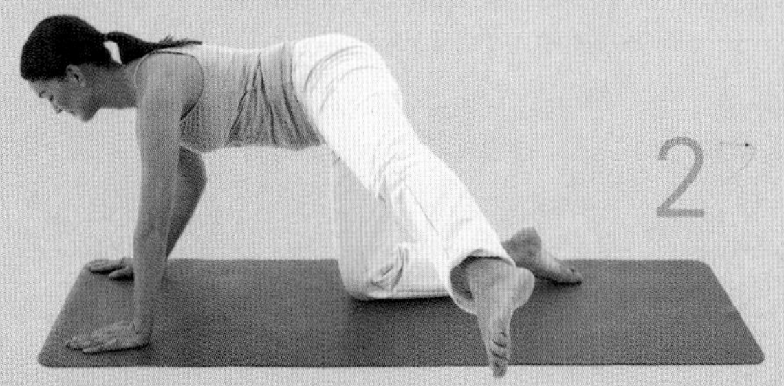

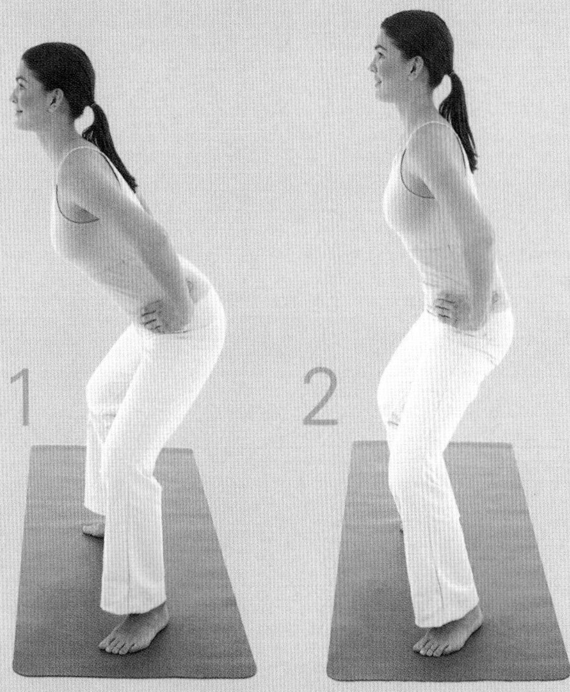

5 Plié 3

1 Stand with your legs hip-width apart and your feet slightly turned out from the hips. Now do a three-count move. First, bend your knees and tilt your pelvis back so that your bottom is sticking out behind you – it should not drop between the legs as in a normal plié.

2 Second, squeeze your buttocks sharply, contract your stomach and press your hips forwards so that your pelvis is now between your legs.

3 Third, slowly straighten your knees so that you return to the starting position.

Repeat this three-count move 10 times, rest, then repeat again
Focus Toning: all buttock muscles, plus hip flexors

5

6

Bottom and hips

Week 5

1 CV combination 1

Make up a routine that lasts 25 minutes by combining all of the following:

- Hop Marching (see page 60)
- Fake Skipping (see page 62)
- V-Dodges (see page 64)
- Boxers' Jogging (see page 66)

Keep alternating the four different exercises with jogging in between to move into the fat-burning zone.

Focus CV

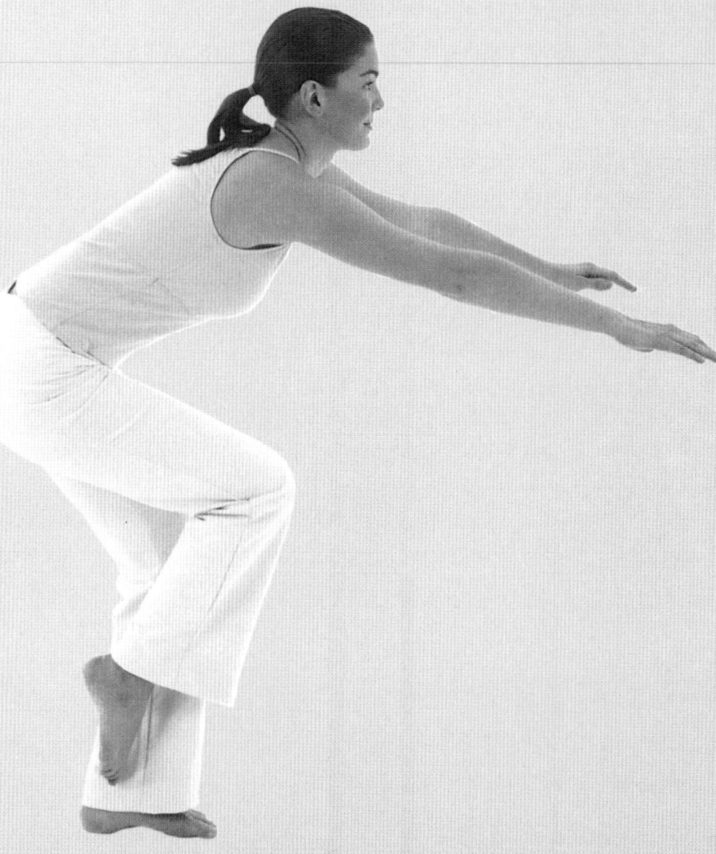

2 One-leg squat

1 Stand with your legs hip-width apart. Pull in your abdominal and pelvic floor muscles. Slowly bend your knees and lower your bottom towards the floor, pushing your bottom and hips behind you. Stretch out your arms in front of you to help you balance.

2 Take one foot just off the ground and hold it for 10 seconds, just touching the other ankle. Shake it out and repeat on the other leg.

Focus Balance

3 Tabletop with weight

1 Get down on all fours, resting on your hands and knees and keeping your back straight. Place a dumbbell securely at the back of one knee and contract the hamstring muscles to keep the weight in place.

2 Keeping your back straight, slowly lift the weighted leg up behind you and back down again. Having to hold the weight really focuses the work on the buttock muscle.

Repeat the lift and lower 25 times, then change legs
Focus Toning: buttock muscles

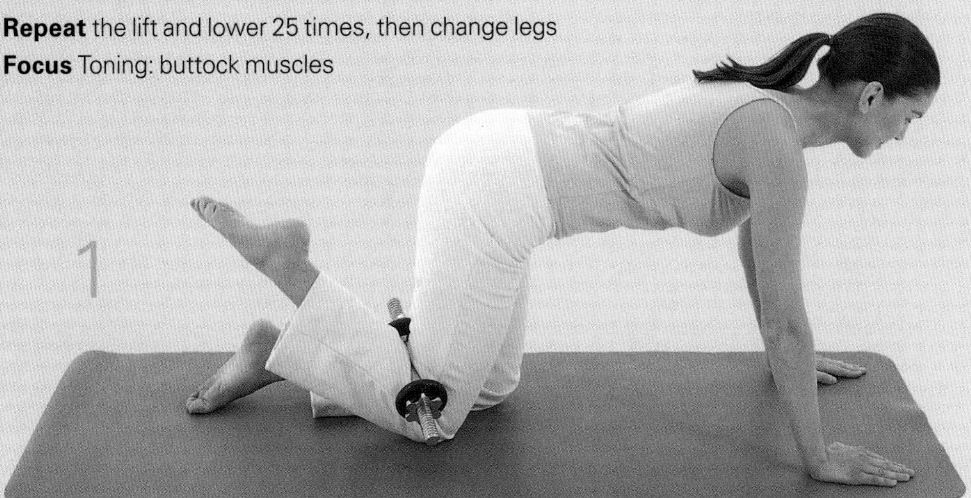

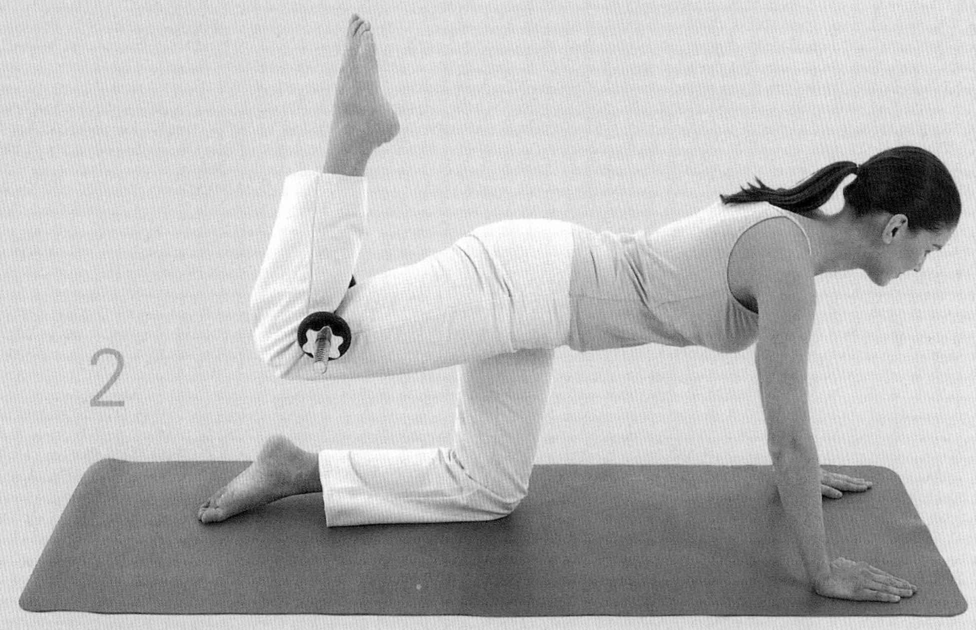

5
6

Bottom and hips

Week 5

4 Tabletop turn-out

1 Get down on all fours (see page 61) but this time extend one leg out behind you with your toes just touching the floor.

2 Now do a four-count sequence: 1– turn the leg out from the hip; 2 – lift your leg up in the air; 3 – turn it back in; 4 – then lower the leg near to the floor. This whole movement must be done without letting your back bow.

Repeat the four-count move on each leg 10 times
Focus Toning: buttock muscles

1

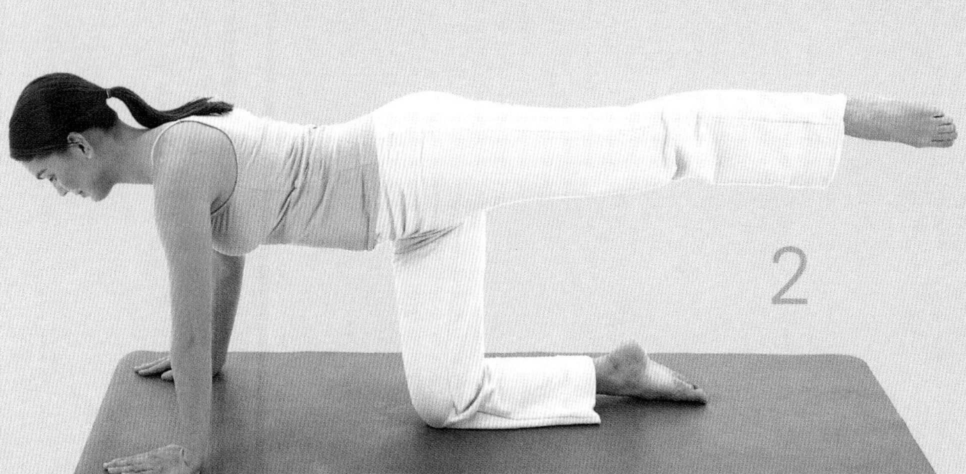

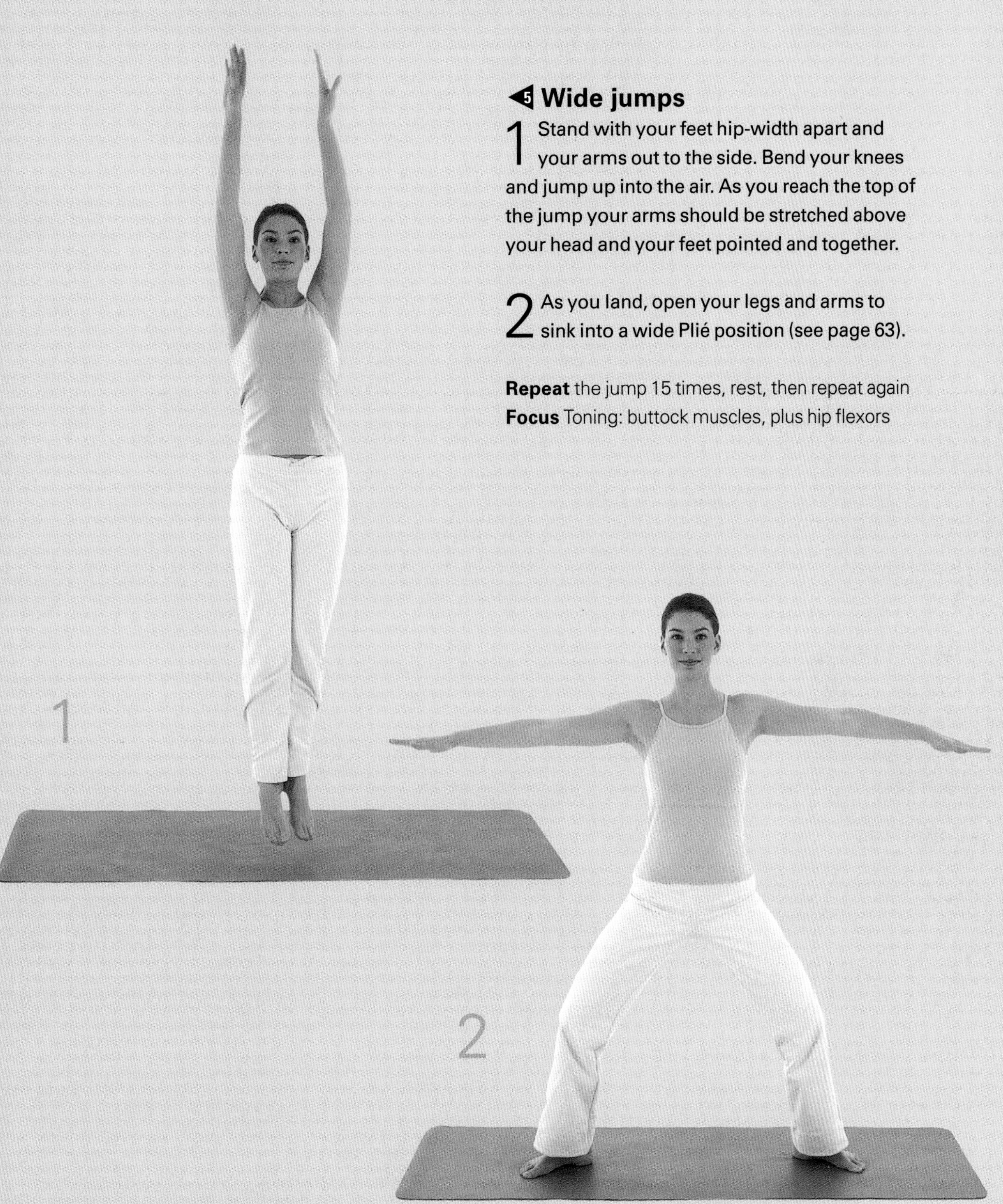

◀5 Wide jumps

1 Stand with your feet hip-width apart and your arms out to the side. Bend your knees and jump up into the air. As you reach the top of the jump your arms should be stretched above your head and your feet pointed and together.

2 As you land, open your legs and arms to sink into a wide Plié position (see page 63).

Repeat the jump 15 times, rest, then repeat again
Focus Toning: buttock muscles, plus hip flexors

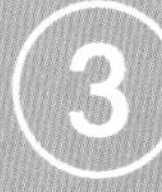

Bottom and hips

Week 6

1 CV combination 2

Make up a routine that lasts 30 minutes by combining all of the following:

- Hop Marching (see page 60)
- Fake Skipping (see page 62)
- V-Dodges (see page 64)
- Boxers' Jogging (see page 66)

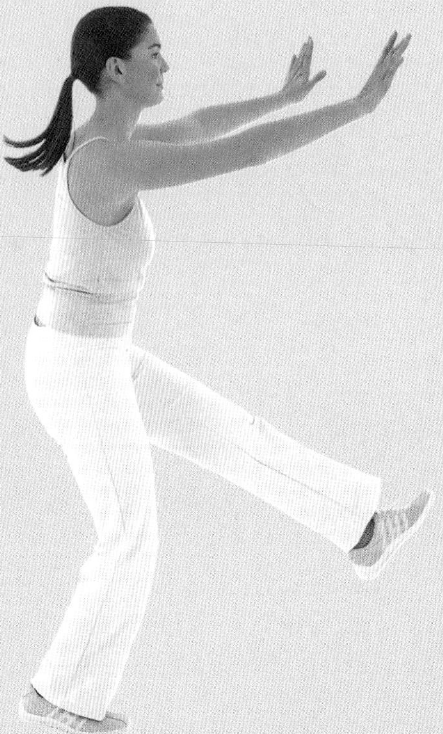

Include the following move to 'up' the pace. This exercise is similar to the Hopscotch move on page 46 but instead of bending the leg up behind you as you jump on to one foot, kick it out in front. Jump on to both feet then jump back on to one foot and kick out. Alternate your feet and do 20 kicks on each leg. If you need to recover, go back to jogging on the spot.

Focus CV

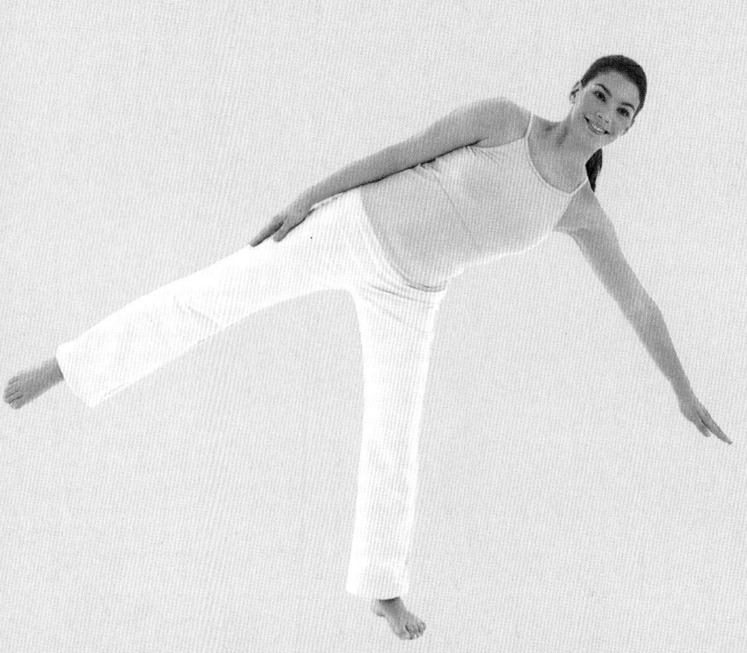

2 Side lean

1 Stand on one leg and take the other leg out to the side. Lift it until it is parallel with the floor. At the same time tilt your upper body to the side until it is also parallel with the floor. Let your arm hang down to the floor in case you lose your balance.

2 Hold this flat-line position for 10 seconds then attempt the same position on the other side. You may find one side is easier to hold than the other.

Focus Balance

3 Attitude lift

1 Stand on one leg and rest your hands on a chair. Now bend the other leg out behind you. The knee is bent and the foot is lower than the knee and the leg should be parallel with the floor. Hold this position until you have it correct. (You should look like a ballerina!) Now just lift and lower your leg slightly.

Repeat the lift and lower with 2 sets of 8 on each leg
Focus Toning: upper part of the buttocks

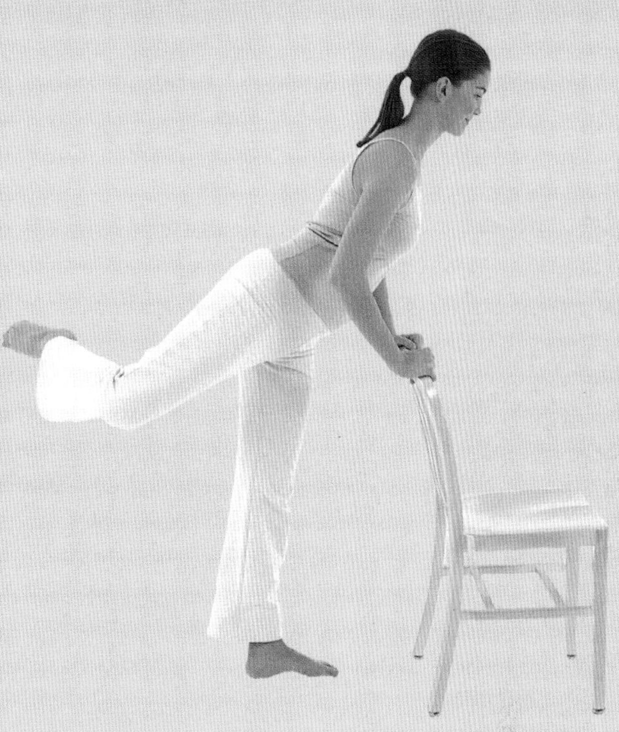

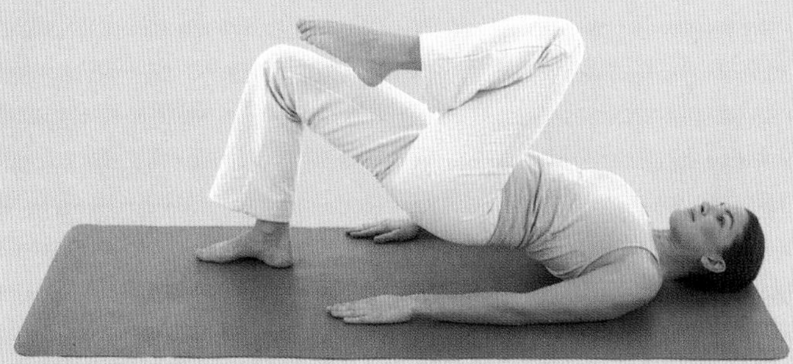

4 Bottom pulse 3

1 Lie on your back and, with one leg in the air, perform one set of pulses from Bottom Pulse 2 (see page 64).

2 Keep your hips lifted but bend the knee right into your chest and do 10 more pulses. Hold still for one breath then do another pulse set of 10.

Repeat the whole of Bottom Pulse 1 (see page 60), 2 (see page 64) and 3 together. Then do the same with the other leg
Focus Toning: buttock muscles

5 Donkey back-kicks

1 Lie on your side, ensuring your hips are aligned one on top of the other. Place both your hands behind your head. Now kick the top leg behind you and bring it back again. The hands behind your head will help you balance as the leg swings behind.

Repeat the kicks 10 times before rolling over and doing the same on the other side
Focus Toning: buttock muscles and hamstrings

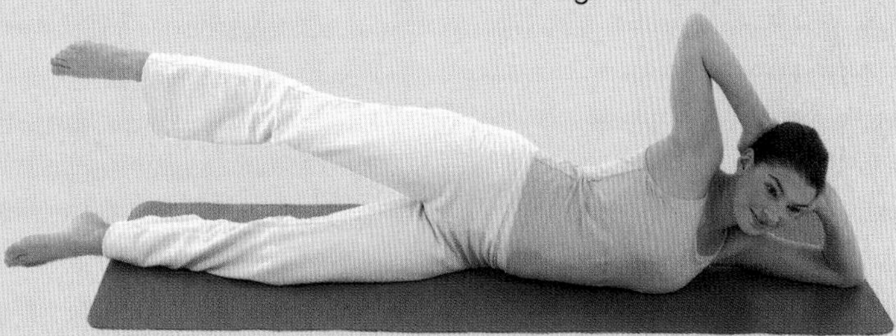

BOTTOM AND HIPS

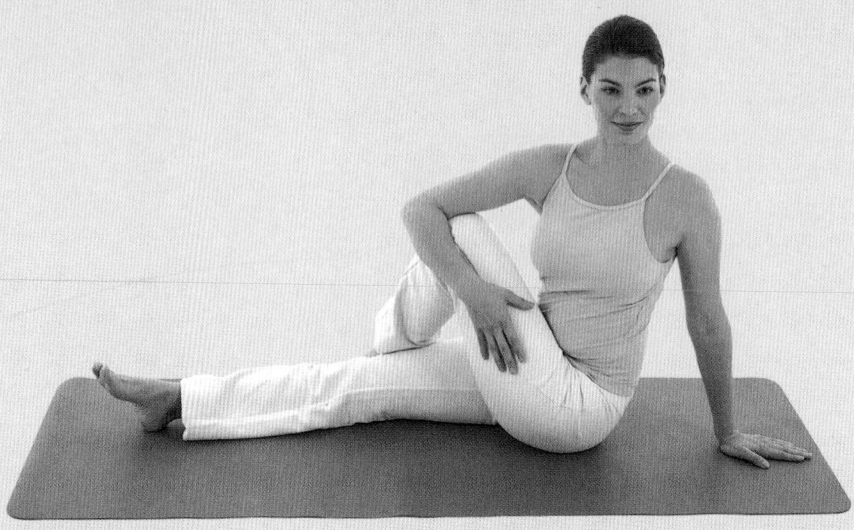

1 Sit and twist

1 Sit on the floor with your legs outstretched. Bend your left leg up towards your chest, cross it over your right leg and place your left foot flat on the floor.

2 Turn your torso towards the knee and wrap your right arm around the upright leg. Pull the knee into your body so that you can feel the stretch in the side of the left buttock. Hold the stretch for 10–15 seconds then release. Repeat on the other side.

2 Sit and lean

1 Sit on the floor with your legs outstretched. Bring your feet towards you so that the soles face each other and your legs are bent to either side of your body.

2 Hold on to your ankles, which should be as near to your crotch as you can get them, and slowly start to lean forwards. Move slowly as you will feel a tightness in the hips. As you lean further forwards you will also feel the top of the buttocks and the lower back start to stretch out. Lean as far forwards as you are able to go, then bring yourself back to an upright position. Repeat once more, leaning slightly further the second time.

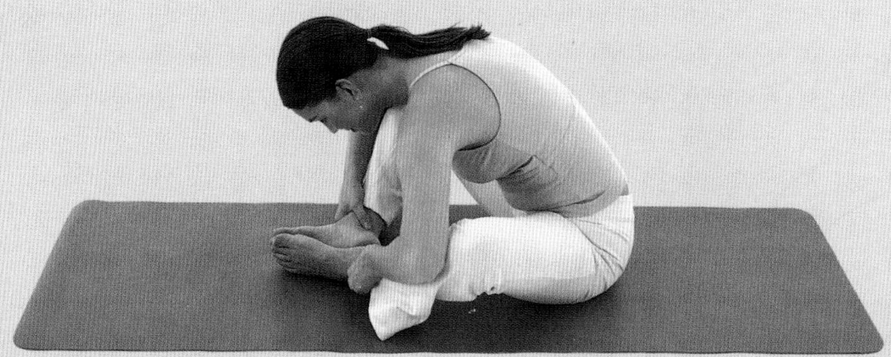

3 Corkscrew

1 Lie on your back with your legs outstretched. Raise your right leg to point towards the ceiling. Bend your left leg and cross it over the right, resting your left foot on your right thigh.

2 Place your hands around your right leg, bend the leg and pull it towards your chest. As you pull the legs towards you, you will really feel the stretch in the left buttock. Hold for 8–10 seconds then repeat on the other leg.

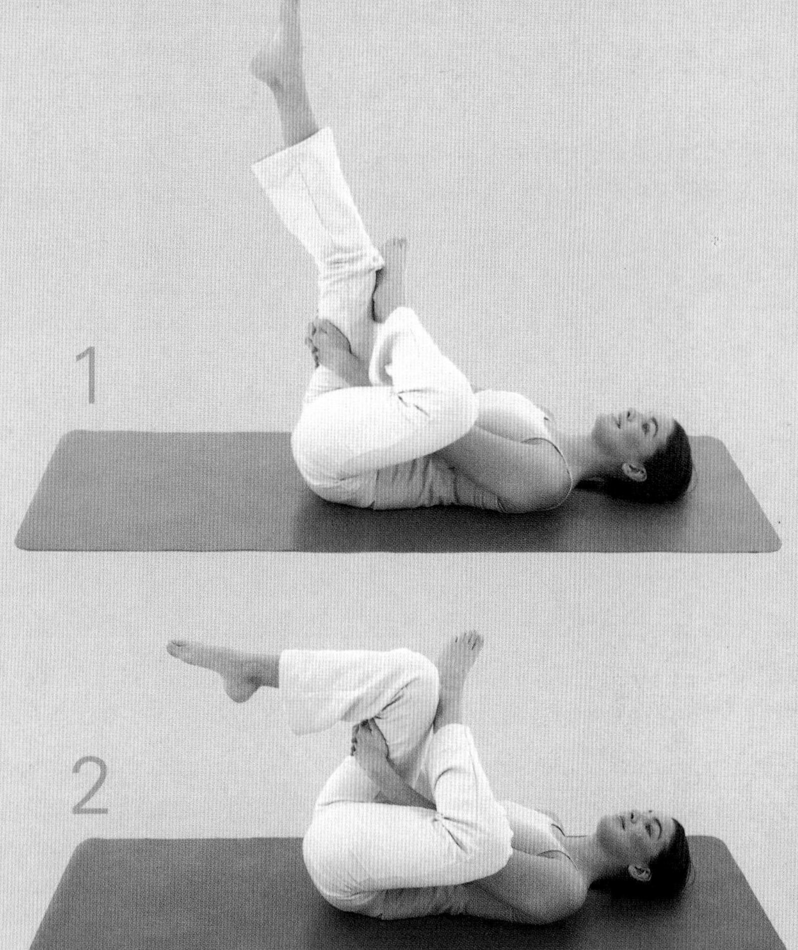

4 Lie and lean

1 Lie on your back with your legs outstretched. Bend your right knee and hug the leg into your chest with your left arm. Stretch your right arm out to the side along the floor to stabilize you.

2 Now pull the right knee towards your left side and hold the position about halfway across your body. Keep the knee pulled tight into your body. You will feel a stretch in the right buttock. Hold for 8–10 seconds then repeat on the other leg.

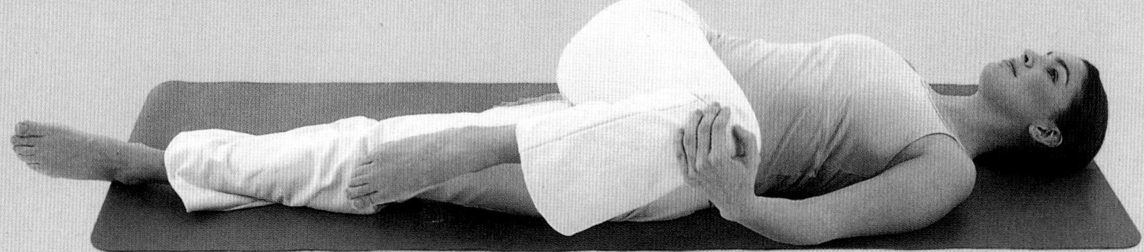

LEGS AND THIGHS

The various muscles in the legs need working in different ways. The exercises aim to cover as many muscles as possible.

Aim to do the legs and thighs exercise routine three or four times each week for the full six weeks for the best results.

Always precede each session with the warm-up exercises below and finish with the stretches on page 92.

Warm-up exercises

These warm-up movements should be performed before each session of legs and thighs exercises to get the blood flowing. Perform these moves as many times as it takes for you to feel warm and really awake – at least 10 minutes. Start by warming up the lower half of the body. Begin by marching on the spot for several minutes to generate some heat (see page 42).

1 Attitude swing

1 Stand tall with your arms out to the sides for balance. Extend one leg behind you, ready to swing the leg forwards and backwards. Keep the swinging leg bent, with the knee turned out and the foot held high. Do not swing the leg too high as you are just warming up the body but swing to the same height front and back.

2 Do 8 swings forwards and back. On the eighth swing hold the leg at the top of the swing – whether it is at the back or the front – for 5 seconds. Pull up in your body and make sure your supporting leg is straight and pulled up. Release and repeat the sequence on the other leg.

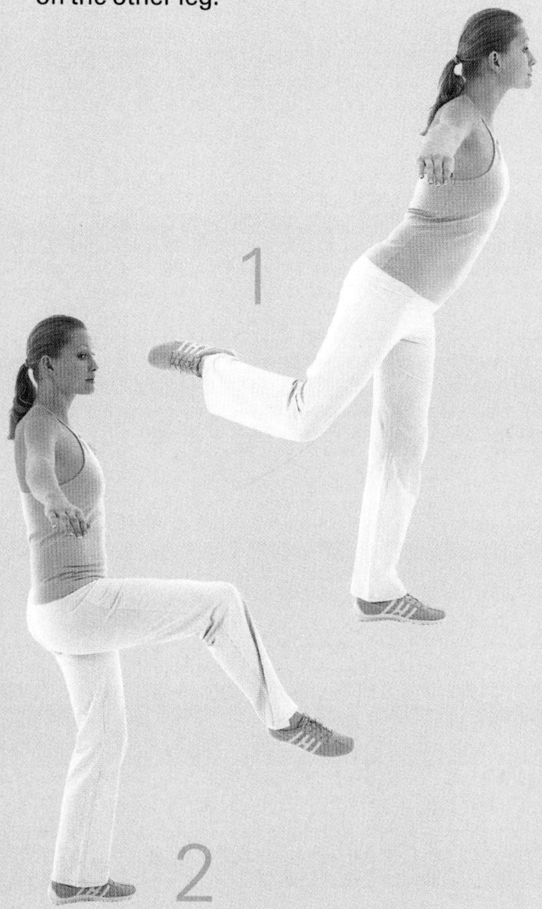

2 Hopped lunges

1 Step into a Lunge position (see page 60). Make sure the knees of your front leg are above your toes but have not gone beyond them.

2 From this lunge position, push off with your legs to jump in the air. Land back into the lunge position and sink down into it. Do 8 push-offs with one leg in front and then repeat with the other leg in front. Rest in between if you need to.

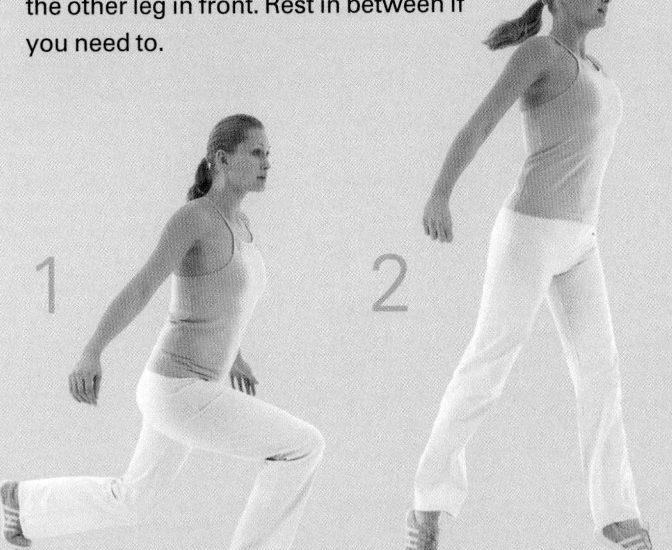

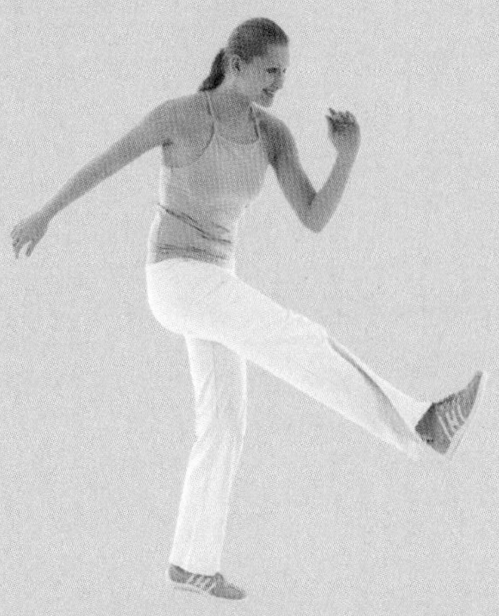

4 Attitude kick

1 Step on to one leg, bend the other leg in then sharply kick it out straight. Continue in this way, stepping on to one leg and then the other to alternate sides. Make the kicks fairly low to start with. As you feel the heat building, start to kick your legs a little higher. You will be getting warm and slightly stretching the back of the legs, most notably the hamstrings. Do 8 kicks on each side.

3 Figure-of-eight swing

1 Stand tall with your hand resting on a chair back and your arm out to the side for balance.

2 Lift one leg and, with it bent, gently move it in a figure-of-eight. First swing the knee in towards the supporting leg then out and around at the front, then swing it back and around at the back to form a figure-of-eight shape.

3 Do 8 to 10 swings to warm up the thigh joint and the legs. Repeat with the other leg.

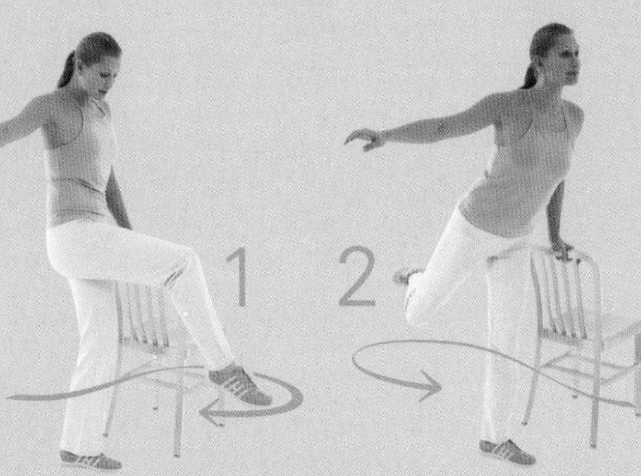

Legs and thighs | Week 1

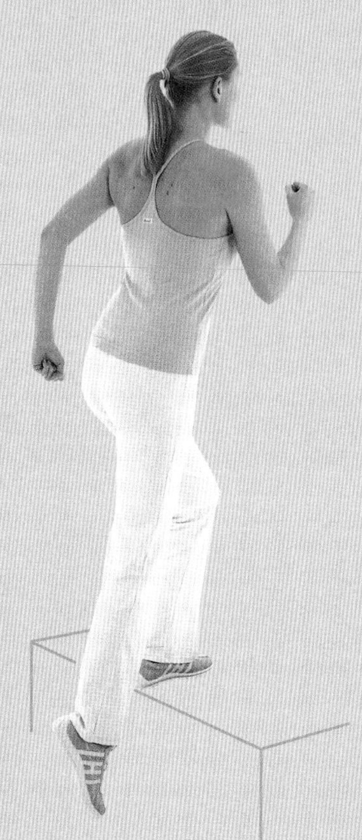

1 Stepping 1

1 Step up and down on the first step of a set of stairs – either at home or in your local park – for 5–10 minutes. Pump your arms as you do this and feel the heat building up.

2 Now step up two stairs at a time and back down again. Change your leading foot every so often and jog up the two stairs and back down. Keep going for 15 minutes.

Focus CV

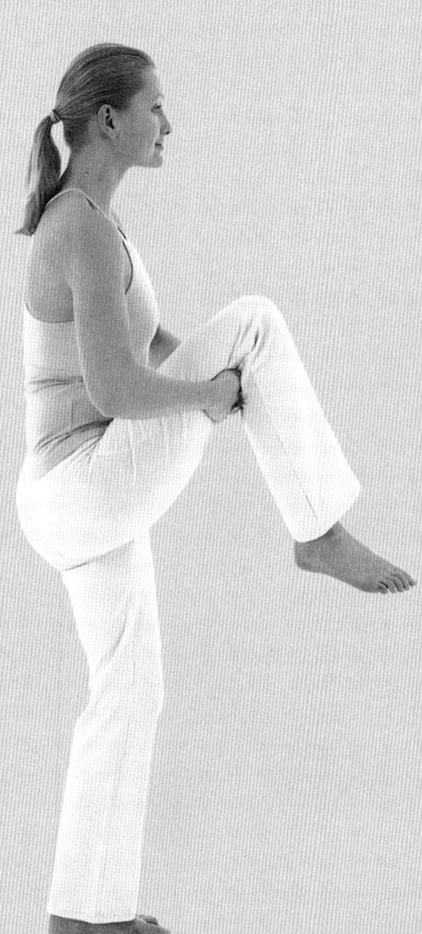

2 Leg hold

1 Swing one leg, with a bent knee, up towards your arms and slip your hands beneath your thigh to catch the leg. Hold this position and balance. Pull up in your abdominals to support your torso and keep your back straight. Try to find a point where the balance is comfortable. Hold for 10 seconds then do the same on the other leg.

Focus Balance

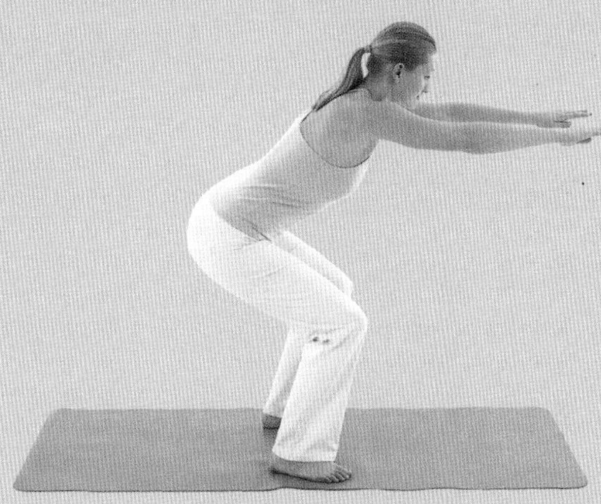

4 Squat 1

1 Stand with your legs hip-width apart. Pull in your abdominal and pelvic floor muscles. Slowly bend your knees and lower your bottom towards the floor, pushing your bottom and hips out behind you as though about to sit down. Raise yourself to standing again.

Repeat squats 8 times, then do another 8, lowering yourself a little further. Rest for 10 seconds before performing a final 8 squats
Focus Toning: all thigh and bottom muscles

3 Seated leg extension

1 Sit on a straight-backed chair and press your hips to the back of the chair so that you are supported in your upright position. Press your knees together.

2 Raise one leg until it is parallel with the floor. Hold the position momentarily, then lower the leg back down. As you tire you will feel the front thigh muscles (quadriceps) starting to ache.

Repeat 20 times on each leg. If this exercise becomes too easy, add some ankle weights and build up to 20 repetitions on each leg
Focus Toning: front thigh muscle

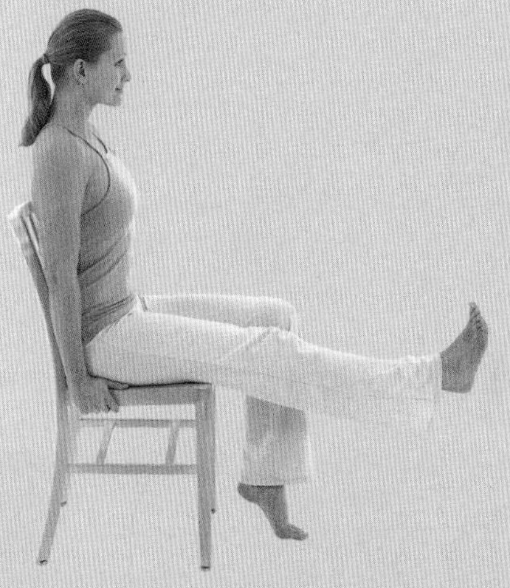

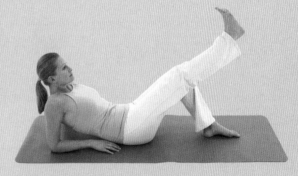

5 Lying leg extension

1 Lie on your back with your knees bent and pressed together and your feet on the floor. Prop yourself up on your elbows.

2 As with Seated Leg Extension (left), extend one leg, hold the position momentarily then bend it back in again.

3 Perform 8 extensions of each of the following; first with a flexed foot; second with a pointed foot; third, while the leg is straight, point your foot, flex it, then point it again. Finish with 8 pointed-foot extensions.

Repeat this whole sequence with the other leg
Focus Toning: front thigh muscles

Legs and thighs

Week 2

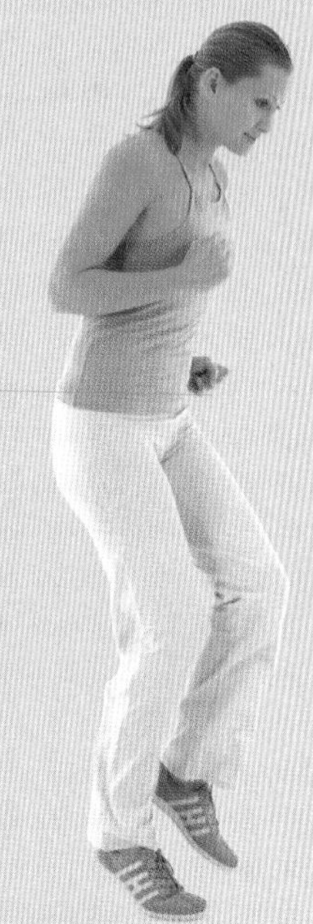

▲1 On-the-spot sprinting

1 Get up on your toes and run on the spot, pumping your arms and moving your legs as fast and as furiously as you can. You won't be able to keep this intensity up for long so alternate this activity with some jogging around the room. Keep going for 20 minutes if possible.

Focus CV

▶2 Quad stretch

1 Stand on one leg. Bend the other leg up behind you, take hold of the ankle and pull your foot into your bottom. Be careful not to swing the hip of the supporting leg out. This move essentially stretches the front of the thigh but also requires a lot of work in the supporting leg to maintain the balance.

2 Hold for 15 seconds then repeat on the other leg.

Focus Balance

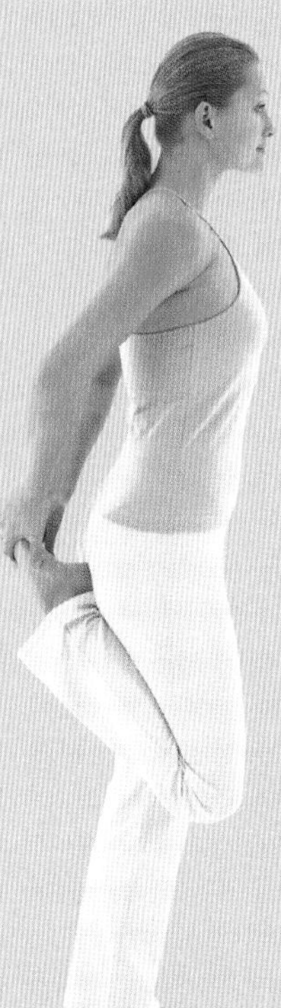

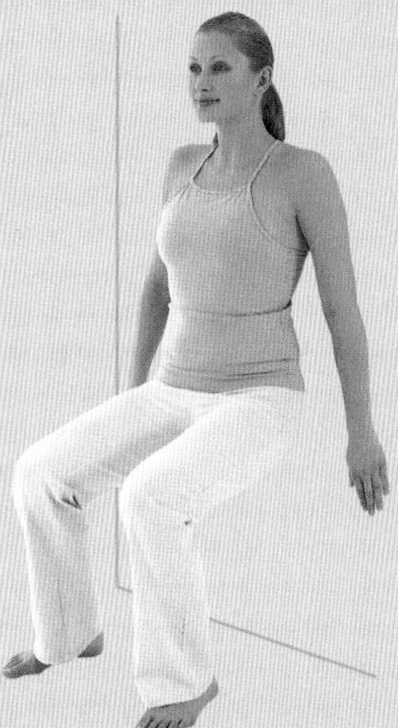

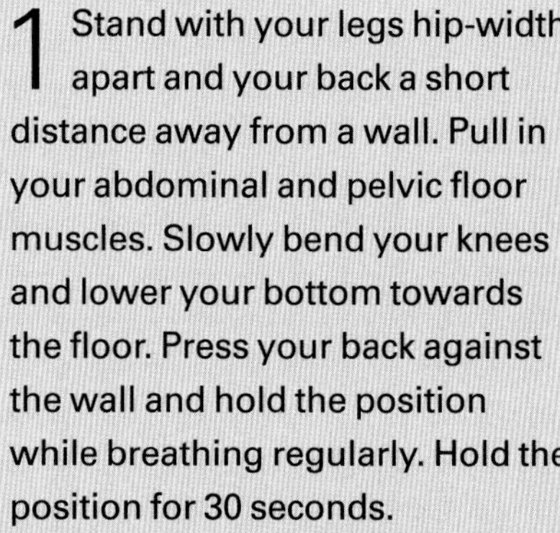

◀3 Squat 2

1 Stand with your legs hip-width apart and your back a short distance away from a wall. Pull in your abdominal and pelvic floor muscles. Slowly bend your knees and lower your bottom towards the floor. Press your back against the wall and hold the position while breathing regularly. Hold the position for 30 seconds.

2 Press upwards again to straighten your legs and then shake them out.

Repeat the hold twice more
Focus Toning: front thigh and buttock muscles

4 Standing leg extension

1 Stand tall with one hand leaning against a wall or chair back to help you balance. Bend the leg furthest from the wall so that the foot is tucked into the other knee.

2 Extend the bent leg out in front of you and hold momentarily. Then bend the leg back to bring the foot into the knee of the straight leg again.

Repeat leg extensions 10 times on each side
Focus Toning: front thigh muscles, plus buttock muscles

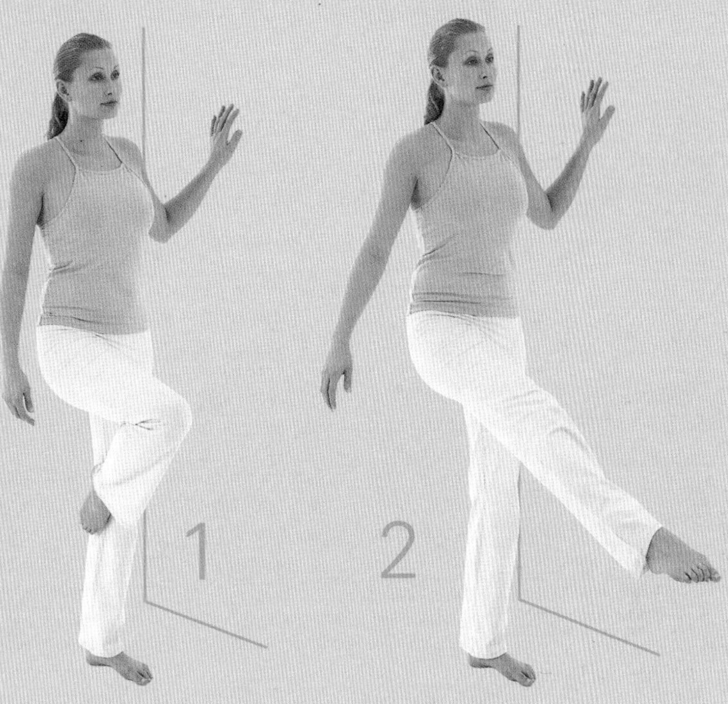

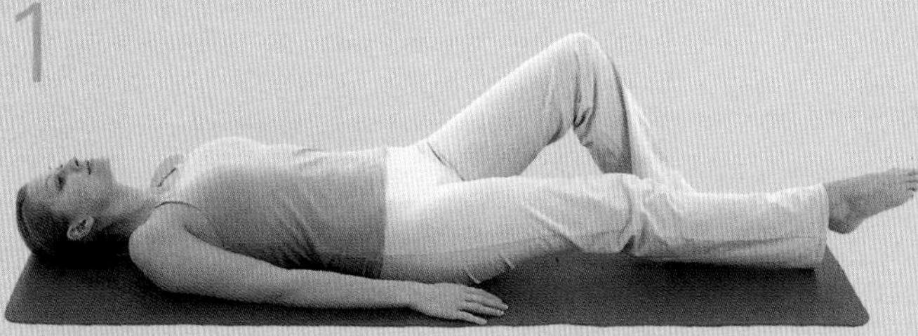

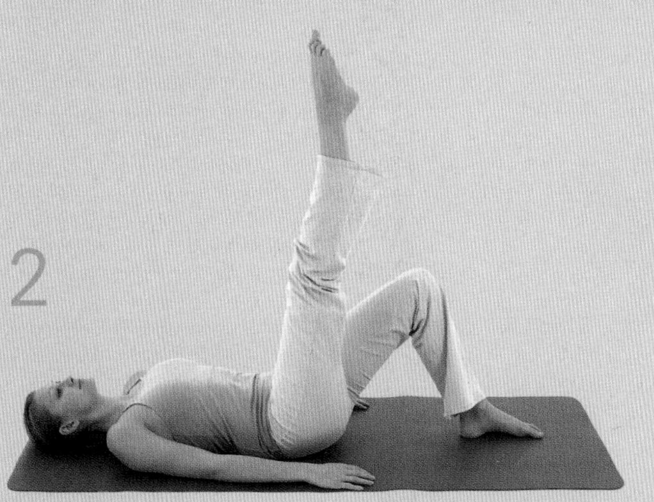

5 Lying leg kick

1 Lie on your back with one knee bent and the foot on the floor, and the other leg outstretched. Press your hands to the floor by your sides. Really extend the straight leg so that it comes just off the floor as you stretch.

2 From this position swing the leg up to the ceiling as high as it will go without hurting then lower it back down with control. The move should have a real swing to it. As your muscles warm up you should be able to swing your leg slightly higher.

Repeat the low swings 8 times on each leg, then 8 higher swings on each leg
Focus Toning: front thigh muscles, plus hip flexors

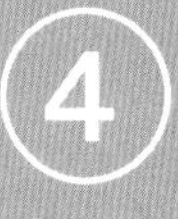

Legs and thighs

Week 3

1 Jogging with star jumps

1 Combine some jogging on the spot and some jogging around the room with Star Jumps – jumping with both feet and arms apart then back in together. The important thing to remember with Star Jumps is to jump high and land softly, slowly bending your knees and lowering your bottom towards the floor. From this bent-knee position spring into the next Star Jump.

2 Do several groups of 8 to 10 Star Jumps interspersed with jogging to get your breath back.

Focus CV

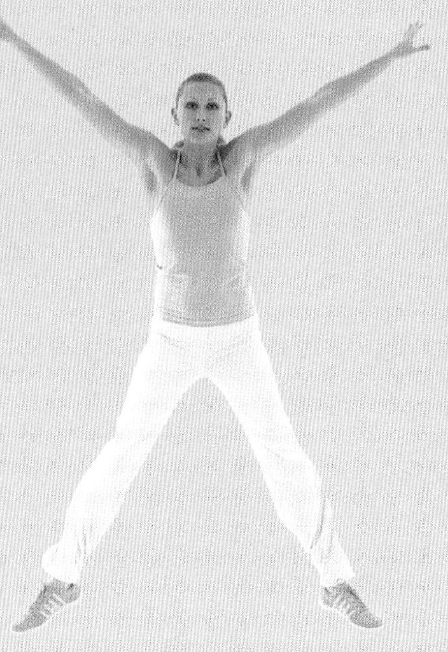

2 Side fall into side lunge

1 Stand with your feet slightly apart and swing one leg out to the side.

2 As you land on this foot, lean into the lunge and hold momentarily before pushing off the foot and returning to an upright position. Perform 8 slow and controlled moves to each side.

Focus Balance

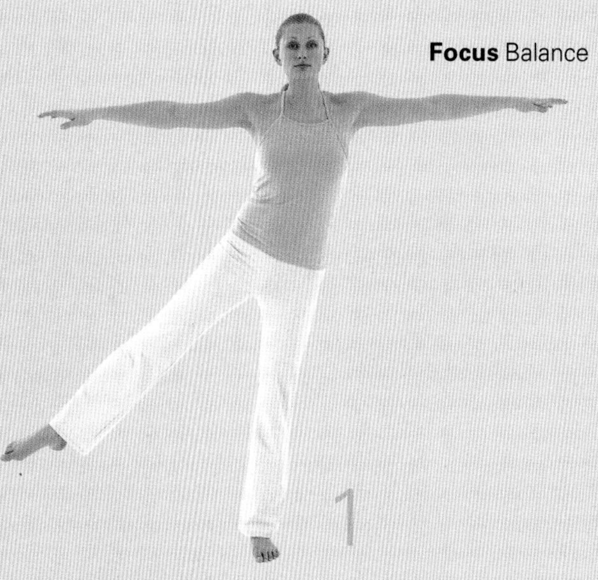

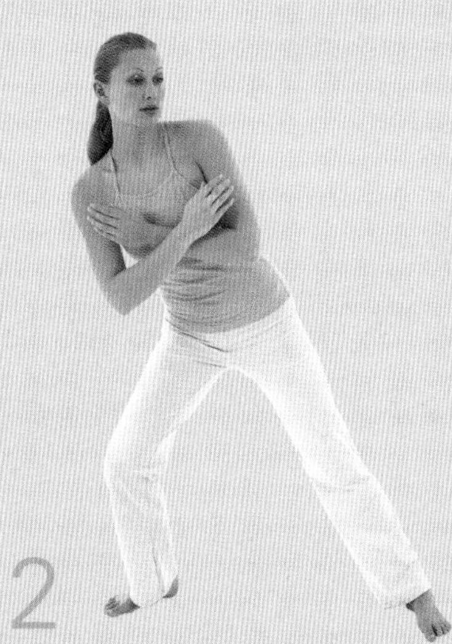

3 Standing side leg extension

1 Stand tall with one hand leaning against a wall or chair back to help you balance. Bend the leg furthest from the wall so that the foot is tucked into the other knee and turn out the leg so that the knee is to the side.

2 Extend the bent leg out to the side and hold momentarily. Then bend the leg back to bring the foot into the knee of the straight leg again. Remember to hold your torso firm – do not let the body sag on to one hip. Also, try not to let the hip on the moving leg hitch up. Keep both hips level.

Repeat leg extensions 8 times on each side
Focus Toning: front thigh muscles

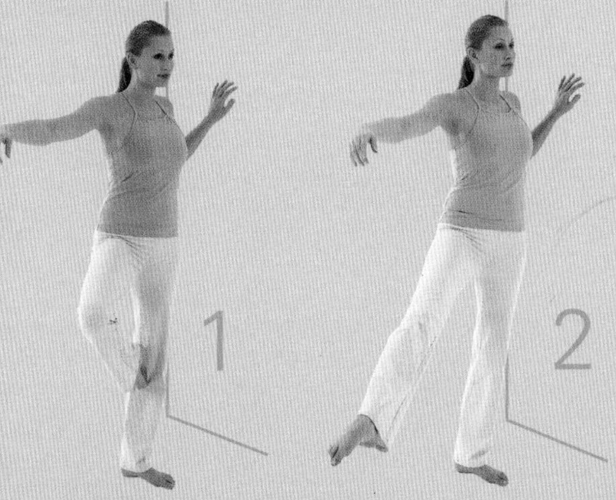

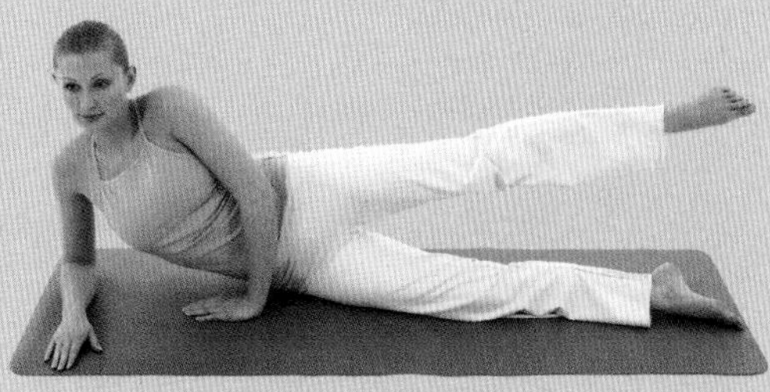

5 Side lifts

1 Lie on your side with one elbow propping you up. Make sure your hips are aligned, one on top of the other, and extend your feet and legs so they are tight and straight.

2 Slowly lift the uppermost leg towards the ceiling as high as it will go. Hold momentarily then lower. If your hips are in the right place, you will only be able to lift your leg to a certain height. If you can get your leg on a level with your ear you have twisted your hips and are not in the correct position.

Repeat lifts 8 times on each leg
Focus Toning: outer thigh muscles

4 Heel raises 1

1 Stand with your feet hip-width apart and your abdominals pulled up and in. Slowly raise your heels off the ground, transfer your weight on to the balls of your feet and rise up until you are fully on tiptoe. Try not to fall off your toes – feel the work through your calves and ankles as you maintain your balance by pulling up through your entire body. Slowly lower your heels.

Repeat rises and lowers 8 times, then give your feet a shake and repeat again
Focus Toning: calf muscles

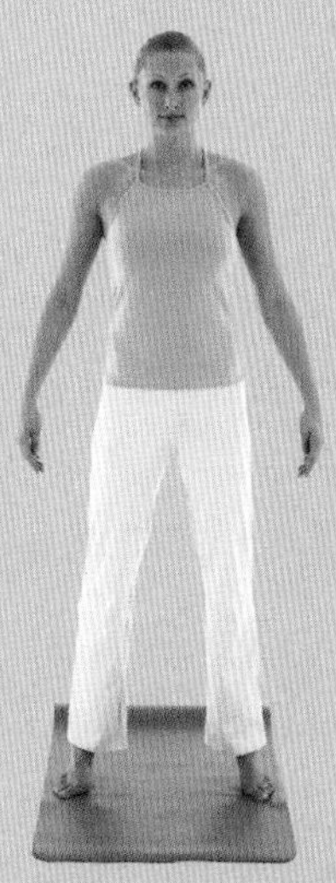

Legs and thighs | Week 4

1 Stepping 2

1 Run up and down a set of stairs – either at home or in your local park. As you come down the stairs, angle your feet so that you don't slip. Run up and down twice. Then do some Step-ups on the bottom step for 2 minutes (see page 78).

2 Run all the way up and down the stairs again twice then step up two stairs at a time and back down again for 4 minutes. Repeat the whole sequence 4 times.

Focus CV

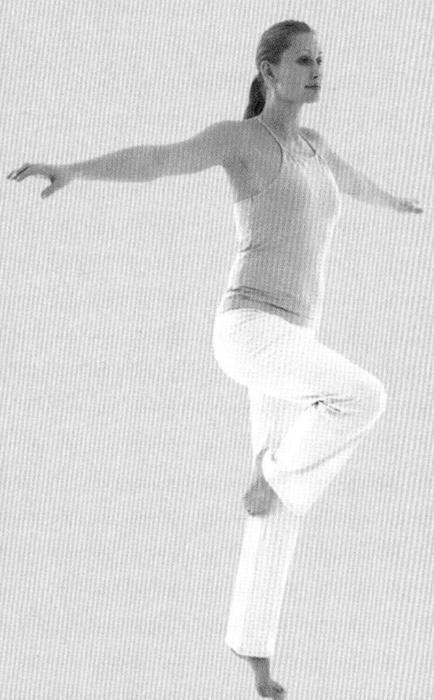

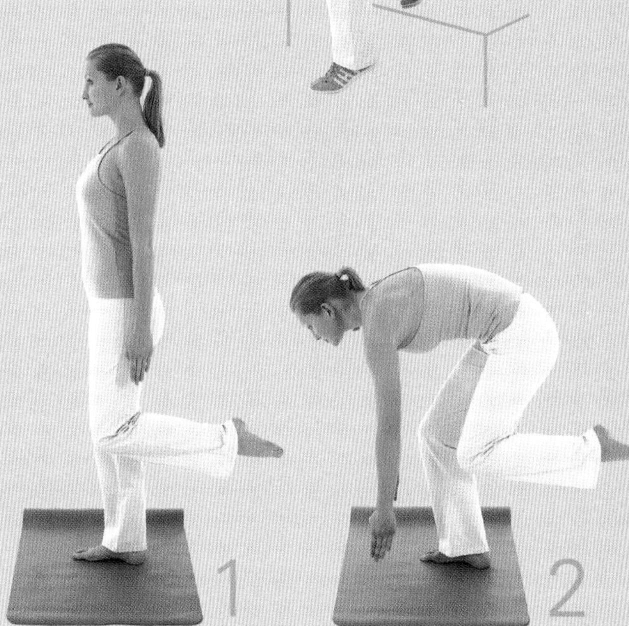

2 Tiptoe hold

1 Stand on one leg. Draw the other leg up to the knee of the supporting leg and hold. Once you are comfortable in the balance try to rise up onto your toes and hold for 8 seconds. Release and repeat on the other leg. Make 3 attempts on each side.

Focus Balance

3 King deadlift 1

1 While standing on one leg, bend the other leg up behind you.

2 Keep your body as upright as possible while bending the knee of the supporting leg so that you can just touch the floor with your fingertips. Push on the leg to straighten up again. This is a tough exercise, which you will feel in your buttocks and thighs. Keep breathing throughout!

Repeat 8 times on each leg
Focus Toning: buttock muscles and front thigh muscles

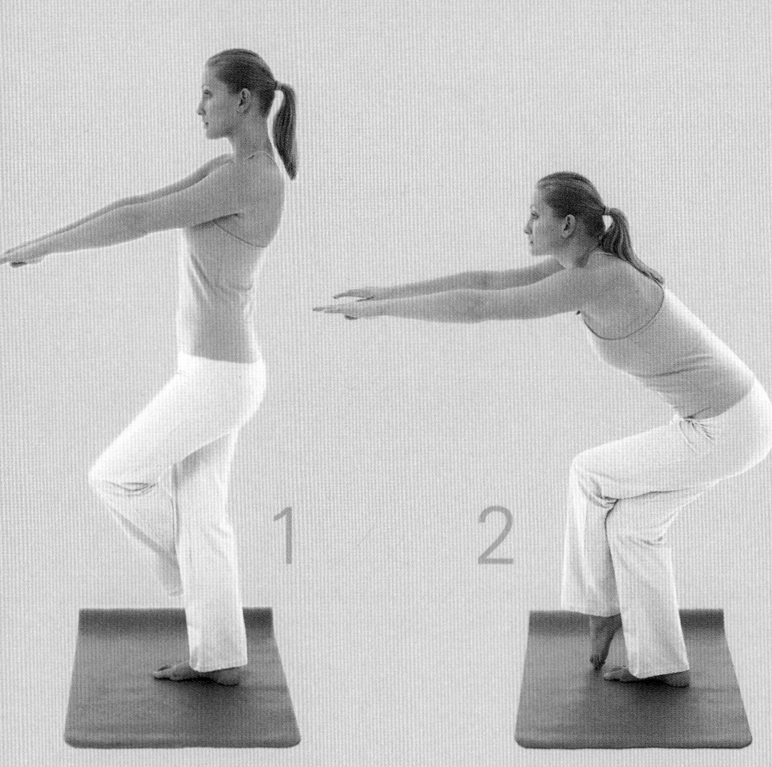

4 Cross-legged squat

1 Stand on one leg with your knee slightly bent. Cross the other leg over the top. Your arms should be extended out in front of you for balance.

2 Bend your knee further until the foot of the crossed leg just touches the floor. Keep your back straight, but tilt your upper body slightly forwards. As you lower your body you will feel this effort on the outside of the thigh and as you straighten you will feel it in the hamstring muscles at the back of the thigh.

Repeat 8 times on each leg
Focus Toning: outer thigh muscles and hamstrings

5 Boot slappers 1

1 Stand with your feet hip-width apart and your hands by your sides. Bend both knees and drop down with your back straight so that you can slap the sides of your ankles with your hands. Push up on both legs to return to your starting position. Alternate between performing this exercise with your heels on the ground (which will work your buttocks and legs) and with your heels lifted when you reach your ankles (which will work the legs and calves more).

Repeat 10 times. Shake out your legs and repeat twice more
Focus Toning: buttock muscles and front thigh muscles

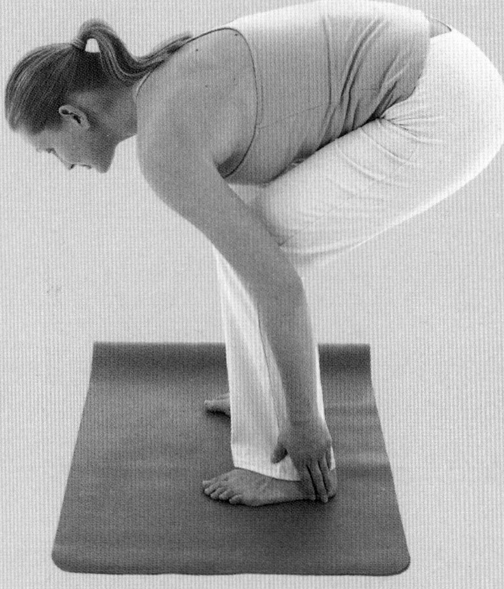

Legs and thighs

Week 5

1 CV combination 1

Make up a routine that lasts 25 minutes. Start with some marching on the spot, build it up to jogging, then intersperse it with:

- On-the-Spot Sprinting (see page 80)
- Stepping 1 (see page 78)
- Stepping 2 (see page 84)

Recover in between the two stepping exercises by marching on the spot if you need to. Finally, step from side to side on the floor to get your breath back.

Focus CV

2 Tip-over

1 Stand on one leg and extend the other leg out behind you. Lift it until it is parallel with the floor. At the same time, lean forwards and let your arms hang down to the floor. Pull up on the thigh of the supporting leg and pull in on your abdominals for support. Hold the position for 5 seconds. Repeat on the other leg.

Focus Balance

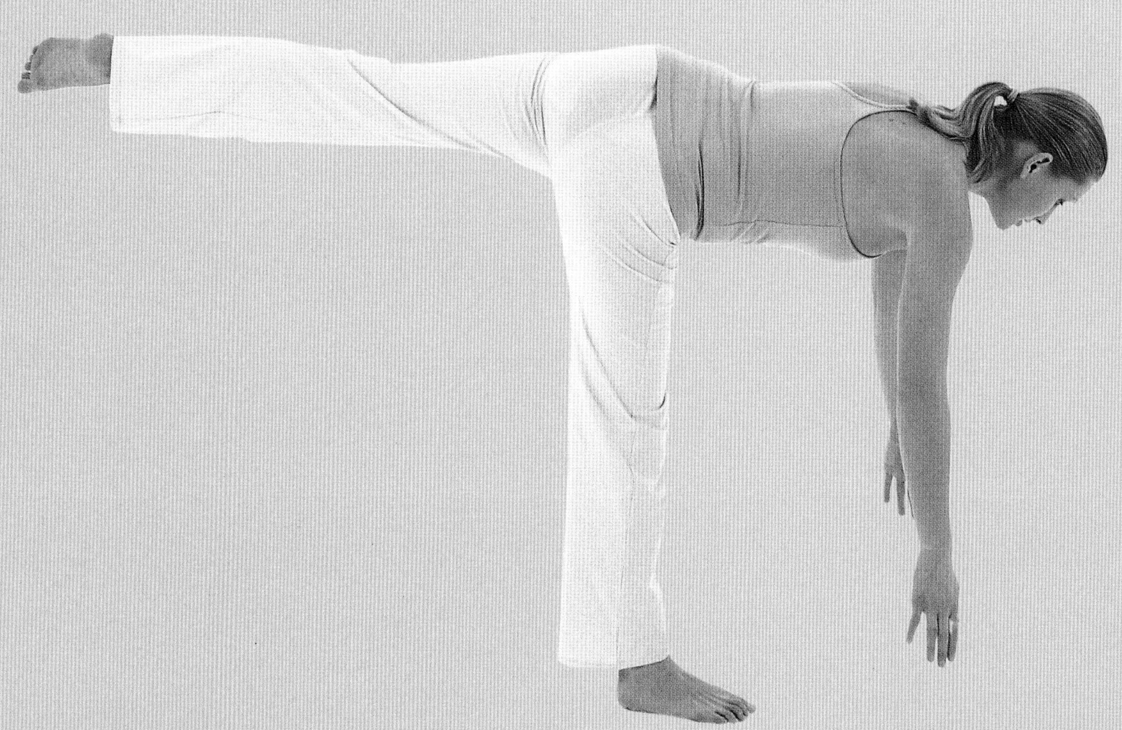

3 Squat jumps

1 From a standing position, bend your knees and lower your hands towards the floor, allowing your heels to lift off the floor.

2 Now push through your lower body to propel yourself high into the air and land by rolling through your feet and bending your knees until you are back into your starting position.

Repeat the jumps 5 times (they are tough!), rest in the squat position, then do 5 more. Take a rest and do a final set of 5, making 15 in all
Focus Toning: buttock and front thigh muscles

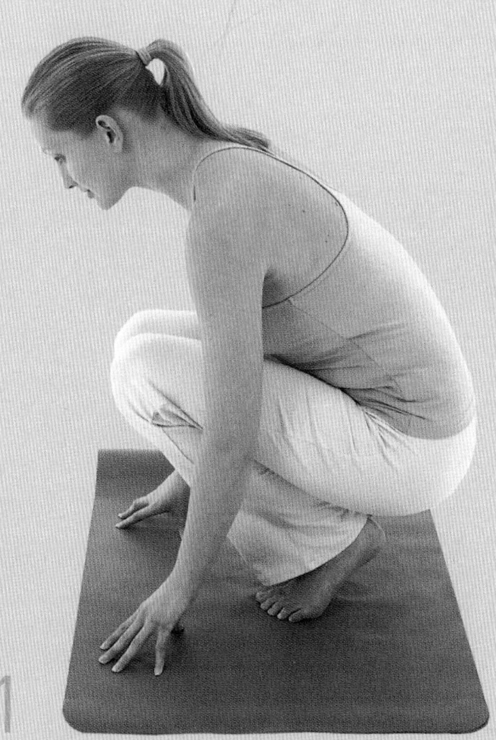

1

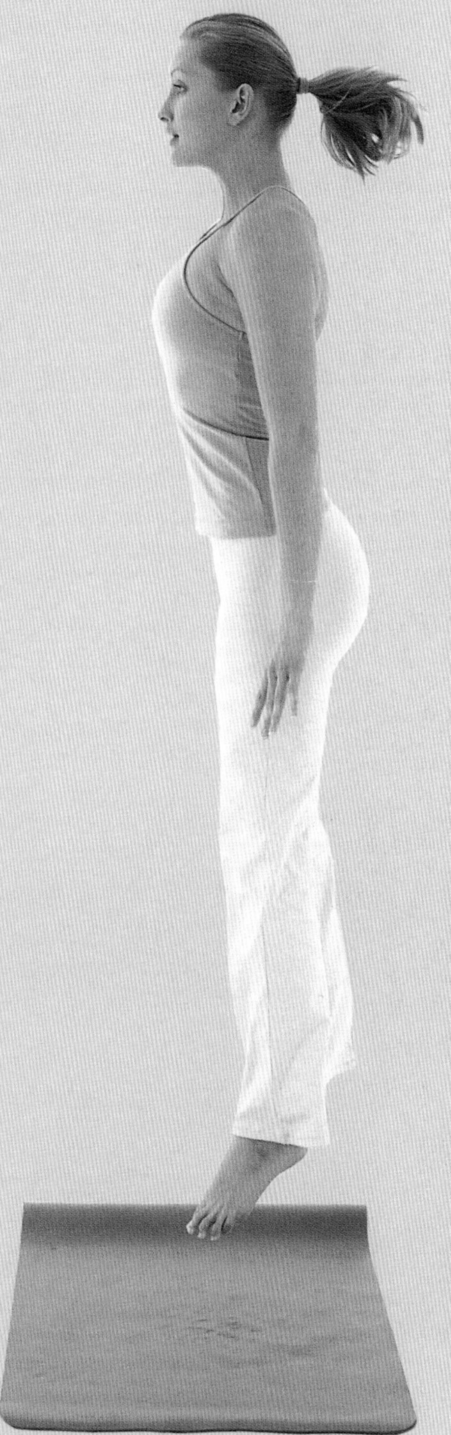

2

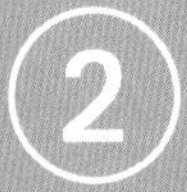

Legs and thighs

Week 5

Leg drawing

1 Lie on your side, ensuring your hips are aligned one on top of the other, and stretch your lower arm along the floor beneath your head. Place your uppermost arm across your body, on to the floor to help you balance. Press your thighs together and lift both legs just off the floor.

2 Turn the top leg out as you slowly bend it and, as though holding a pencil with your big toe and drawing a line, slide your foot all the way up the bottom leg until it comes to the knee. Slowly slide the leg back down until it is straight again. Remember to keep breathing regularly throughout this exercise.

Repeat 8 times on each leg, rolling over to change sides
Focus Toning: inner thigh muscles

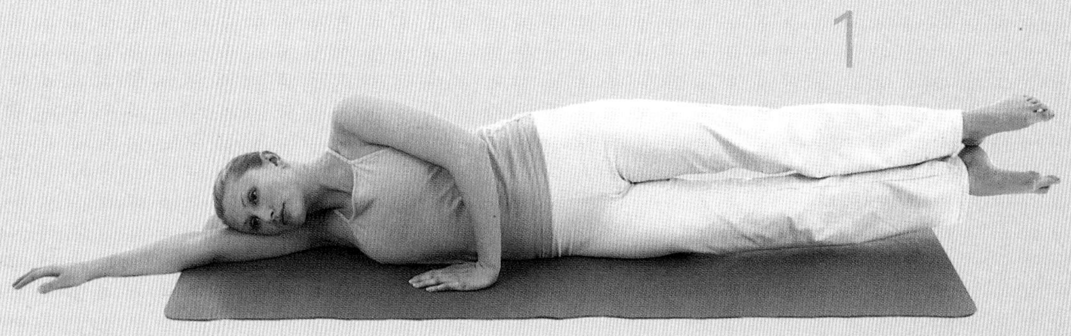

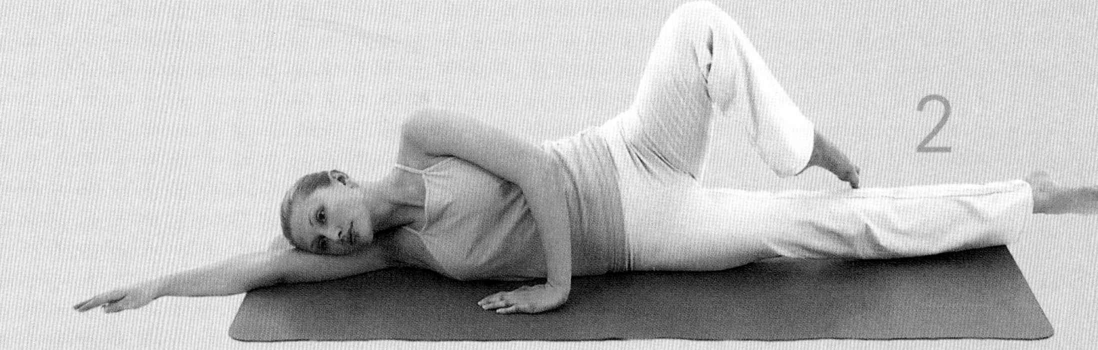

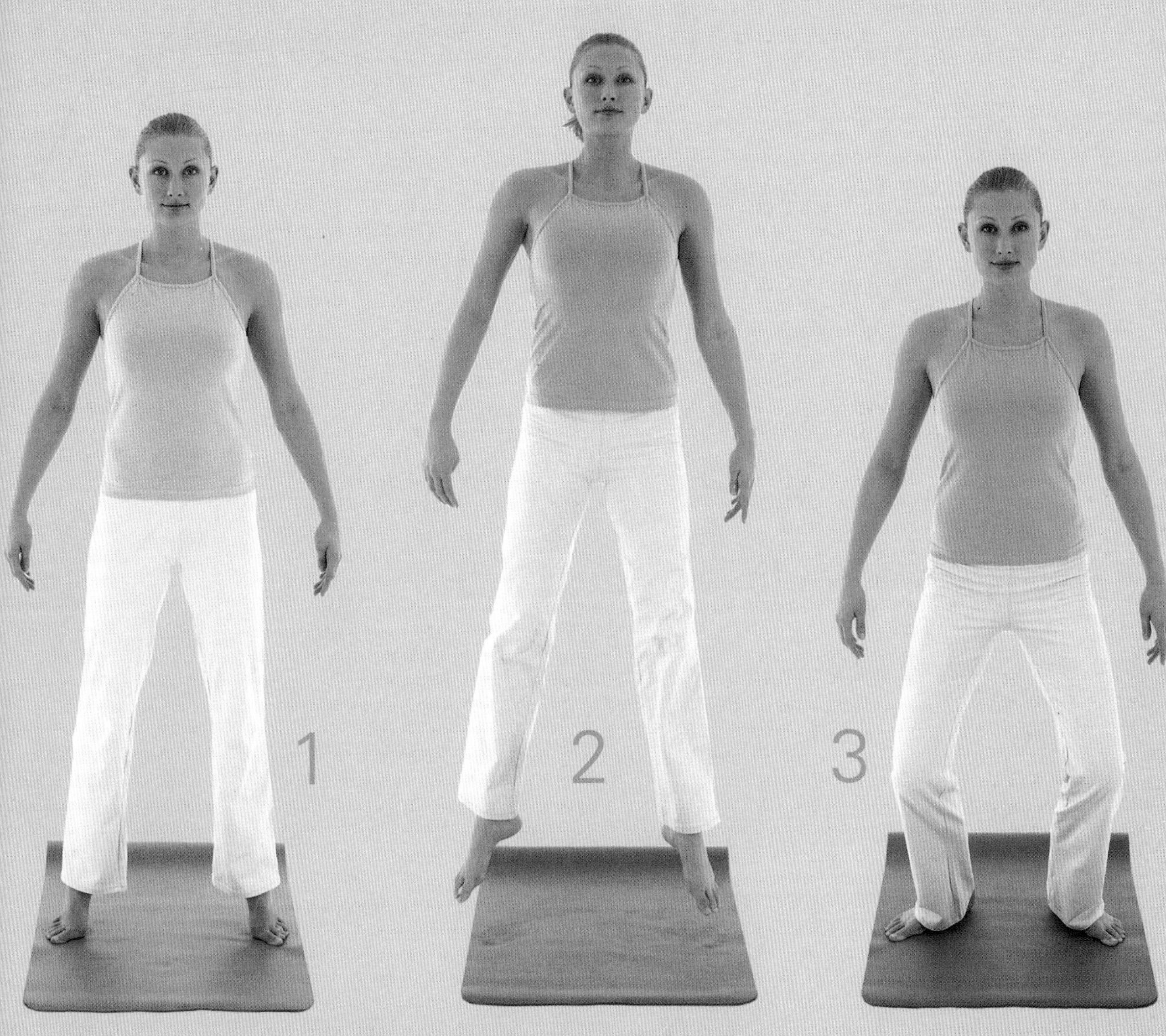

5 Heel raises 2

1 Raise yourself onto your toes as in Heel Raises 1 (see page 83).

2 Now bend your knees and push up and spring off your toes into a jump.

3 As you land, bend your knees softly and with control before pushing off again. Keep your body as upright as you can with your bottom tucked under as you softly bend your knees.

Repeat jumps 15 times, rest, then repeat again
Focus Toning: calf muscles

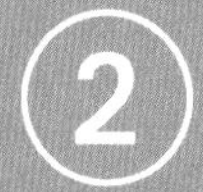

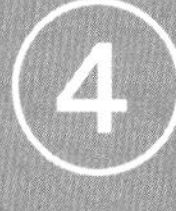

6

Legs and thighs

Week 6

1 CV combination 2

Make up a routine that lasts 30 minutes by combining all of the following:

- Stepping 1 (see page 78)
- On-the-Spot Sprinting (see page 80)
- Jogging with Star Jumps (see page 82)
- Stepping 2 (see page 84)

Include the balance exercise, Side Fall into Side Lunge (see page 82) after each CV exercise. If you need to recover, go back to jogging on the spot.

Focus CV

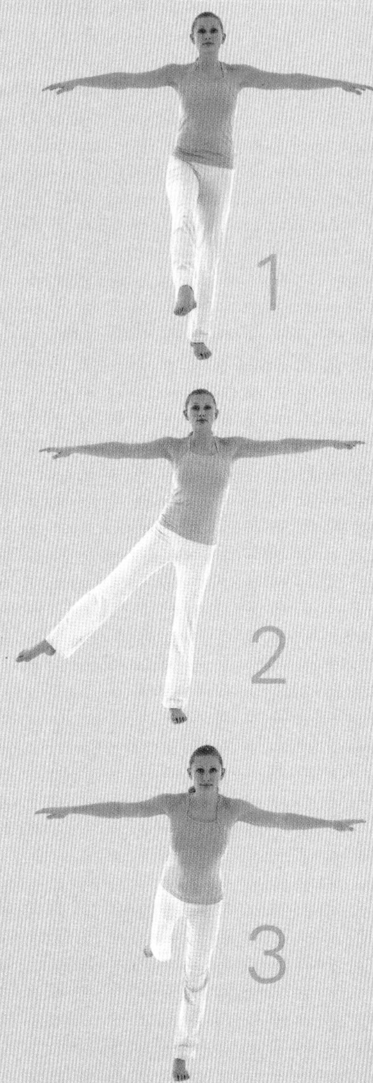

2 The cross

1 Stand on one leg. Bring the other foot up until it touches the supporting knee. Hold your arms out to the side and pull in your abdominals to help you balance. Extend your leg out to the front, then pull your foot back into the knee.

2 Turn your knee out to the side, extend your leg out and then pull your foot back into your knee.

3 Lastly, push your leg out behind you then bring it back in again. These three moves, extending the leg in each direction, should be done without losing your balance! Pull up on your supporting leg throughout and keep breathing.

Focus Balance

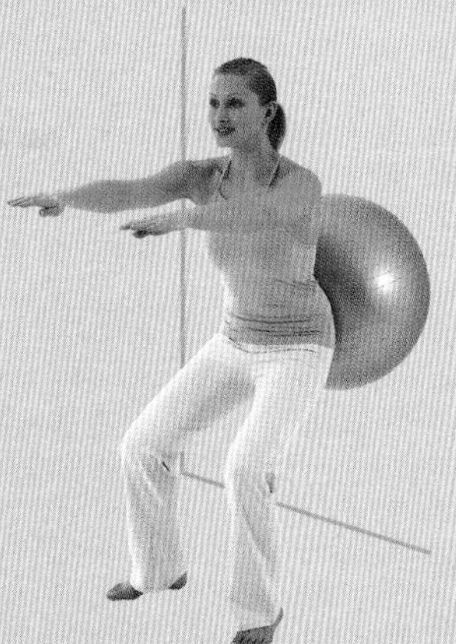

3 Squat with ball

1 Stand with your legs hip-width apart and place the ball behind your upper back. Slowly bend your knees and lower your bottom towards the floor, pushing your bottom and hips behind you to press the ball against the wall. Raise yourself by rolling the ball up the wall to standing again.

Repeat bends 8 times
Focus Toning: buttock and front thigh muscles

▼4 King deadlift 2

1 Stand on one leg and extend the other leg out behind you. Hold one arm out for balance and place the hand of the other on a wall for support.

2 Slowly try to bend the knee of the supporting leg, using the wall to help you. Lower yourself until the knee is fully bent then attempt to straighten up again. Always contract and use your abdominals to support your torso.

Repeat 3 times on each leg
Focus Toning: buttock and front thigh muscles

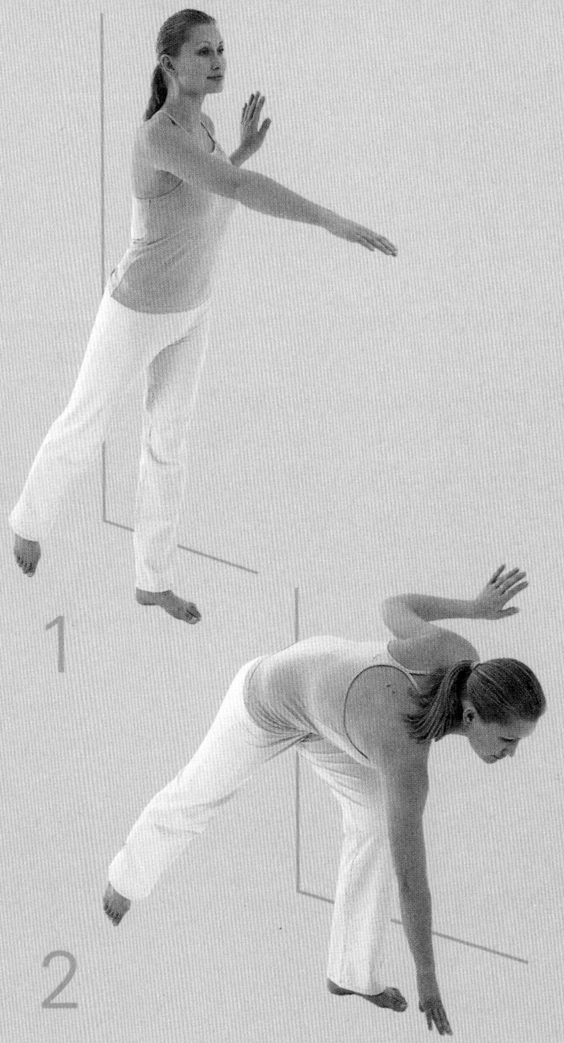

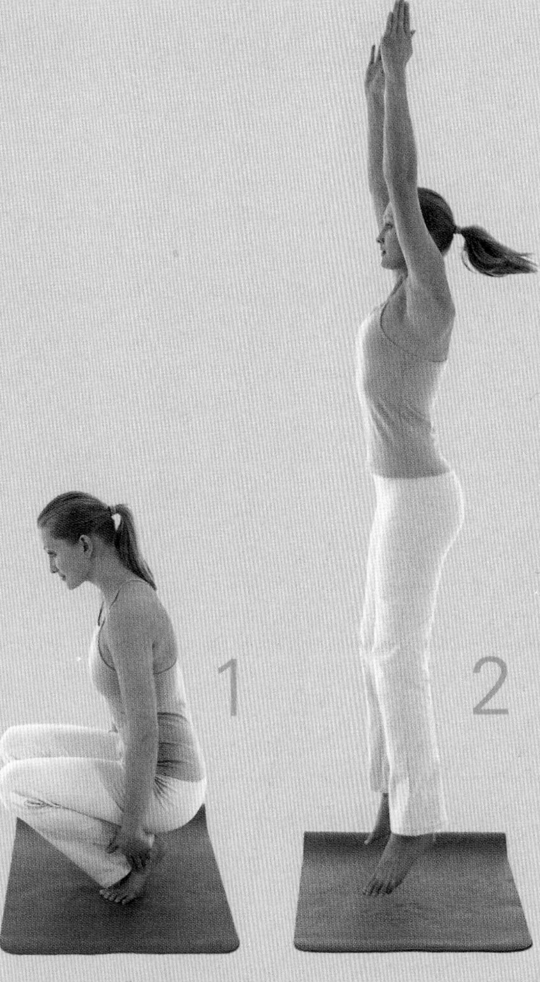

▲5 Boot slappers 2

1 Stand with your feet hip-width apart and your hands by your sides. Keeping your heels on the floor, bend both knees and drop down with your back straight so that you can slap the sides of your ankles with your hands.

2 Push up on both legs and jump up. Land with your knees bent before you drop to repeat the move.

Repeat 10 times. Shake your legs out and repeat twice more
Focus Toning: buttock and front thigh muscles

LEGS AND THIGHS

1 First stretch

1 Sit as tall as you can with your legs outstretched and your feet flexed. Lean forwards and stretch your arms towards your feet. Aim to press forward from the bottom of your back so as to feel the stretch in your back as well as in your hamstrings.

2 Second stretch

1 Sit with your legs out to the sides and place your hands on the floor in front of you. Gently walk your hands along the floor away from you, pulling your chest towards the floor. You will feel this stretch along your inner thighs and hamstrings. Reach as far as you can where it still feels comfortable, hold the position, then walk your hands a little further forward.

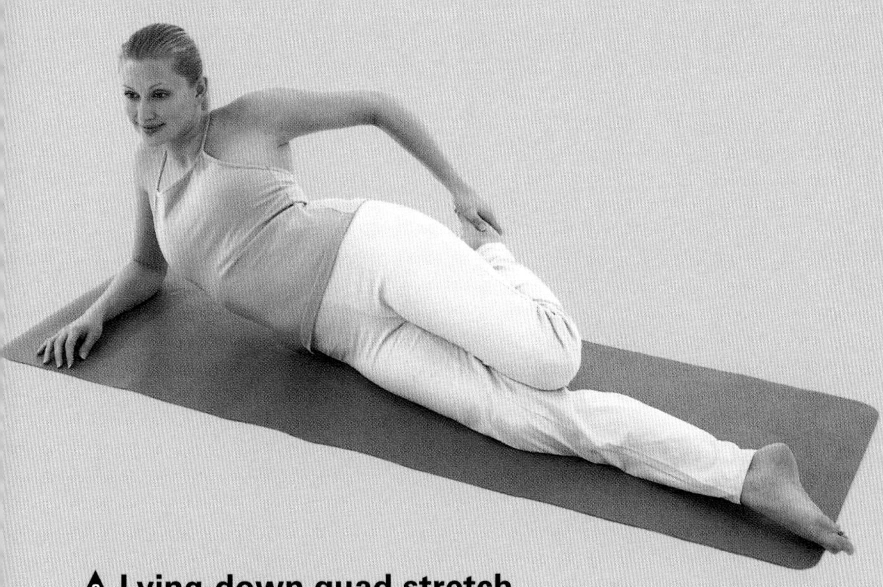

3 Lying-down quad stretch

1 Lie on your side with one elbow propping you up. Make sure your hips are aligned, one on top of the other. Bend the uppermost leg behind you, taking hold of the ankle with one hand. Pull your foot in towards your bottom and hold the position for 15 seconds – you will feel the stretch in the front of the thigh. To increase the stretch, pull in your abdominals and push your hips forwards. Roll over and repeat the stretch on the other leg.

4 Splits

1 Step forwards into a Lunge position (see page 60) but drop much lower. Place your hands on the floor either side of the bent front knee.

2 Now drop the back knee and place the top of the foot on the floor. From here simply slide the back leg away from the front leg as far as you can until you are doing 'the splits'. It doesn't matter if you cannot go this far – just push the back leg away as far as you can. Once you get to your limit, stay there and hold for a few seconds, then repeat the exercise on the other leg.

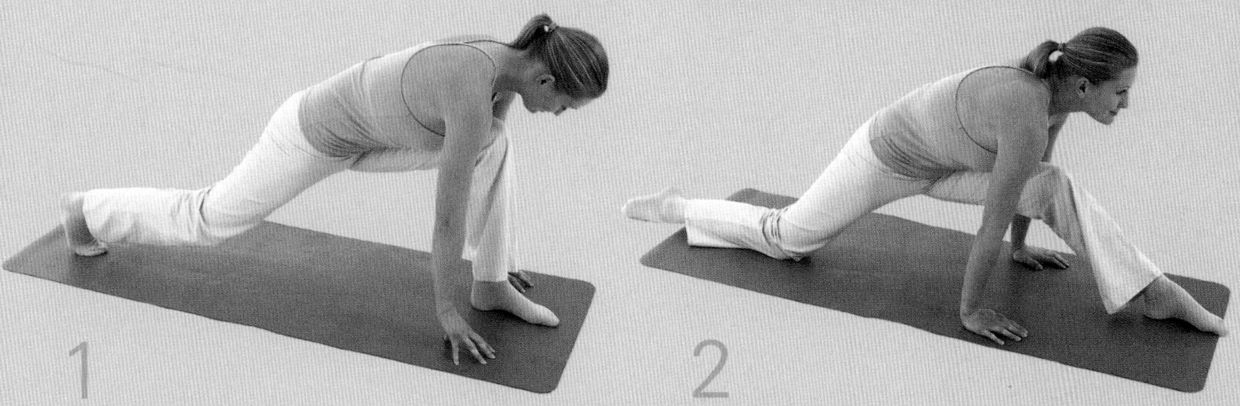

ARMS AND UPPER BODY

Aim to do the arms and upper body exercise routine three or four times each week for the full six weeks for the best results.

Always precede each session with the warm-up exercises below and finish with the stretches on pages 110–111.

Warm-up exercises

These warm-up movements should be performed before each session of arms and upper body exercises to get the blood flowing.

1 Handy circles

1 Stand tall with your abdominals pulled in. Place your hands on your shoulders and try to draw a full circle with each elbow. Do 8 circles one way and then the other. Keeping your hands on your shoulders enables the whole of the shoulder joint to get warm as you rotate your arms.

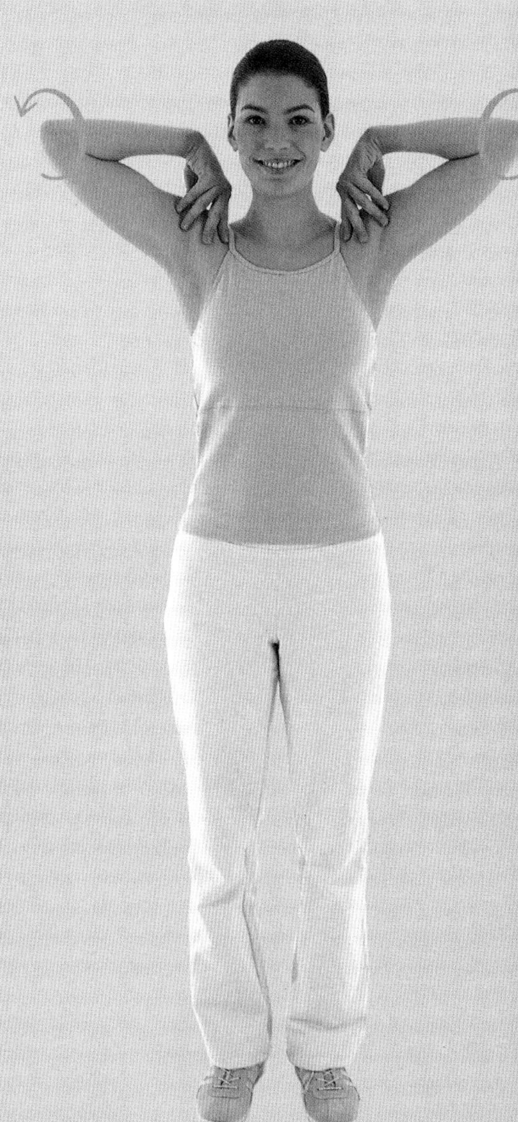

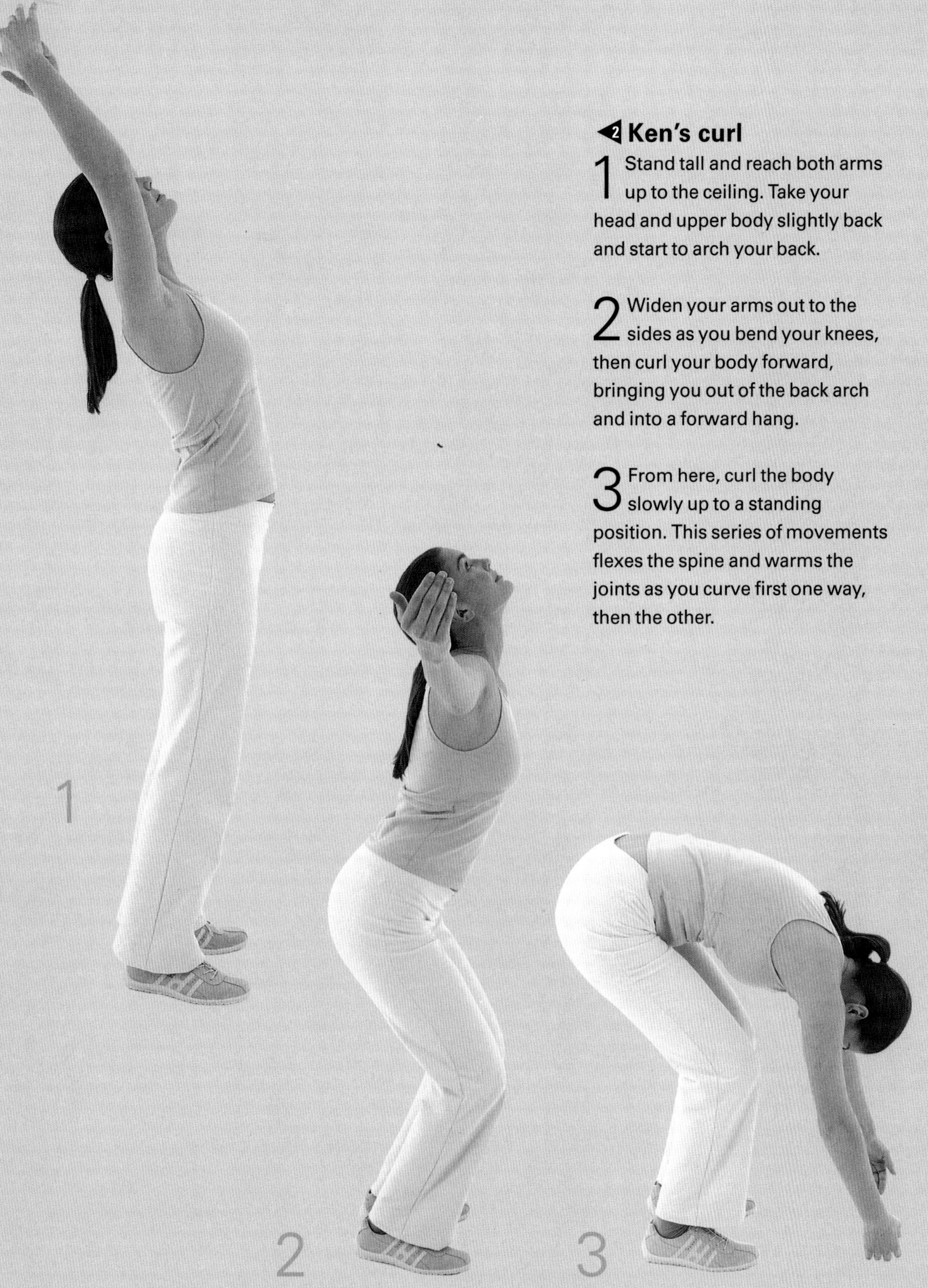

2 Ken's curl

1 Stand tall and reach both arms up to the ceiling. Take your head and upper body slightly back and start to arch your back.

2 Widen your arms out to the sides as you bend your knees, then curl your body forward, bringing you out of the back arch and into a forward hang.

3 From here, curl the body slowly up to a standing position. This series of movements flexes the spine and warms the joints as you curve first one way, then the other.

Arms and upper body

Shoulder shrugs

1 From a standing position, lean forward with your knees slightly bent and let your arms hang down. Gently shrug your shoulders up to your ears and drop them down to generate some warmth in the shoulder area. Do this several times and then slowly curve your spine back to a standing position.

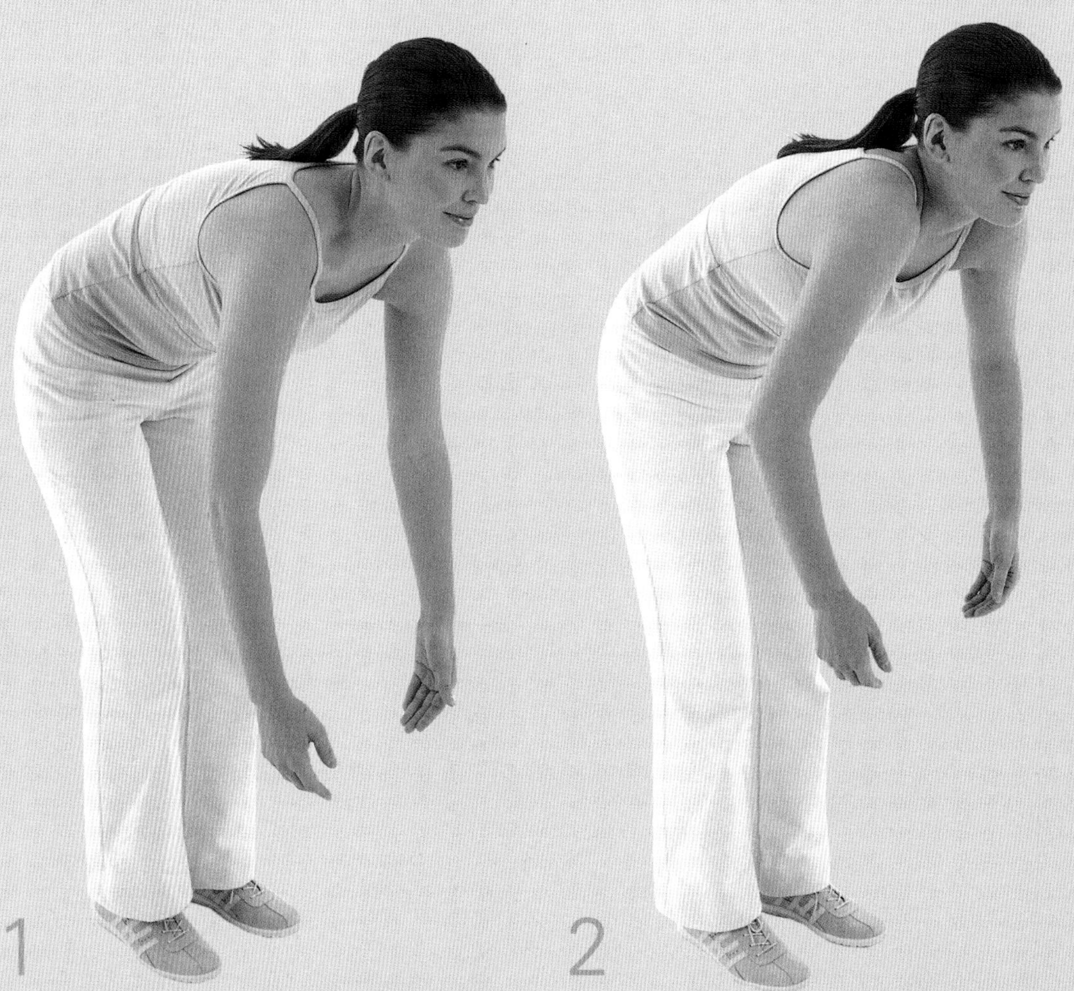

4 Sad cat, happy cat

1 Get down on all fours, resting on your hands and knees and draw in your stomach as much as you can – really feel like you are pulling your navel towards the back of your spine. As you do this, allow your back to arch upwards like a cat.

2 Hold this position then push your spine in the opposite direction so that your back is curved. Keep breathing as you bend the spine first one way and then the other to warm up the whole spine.

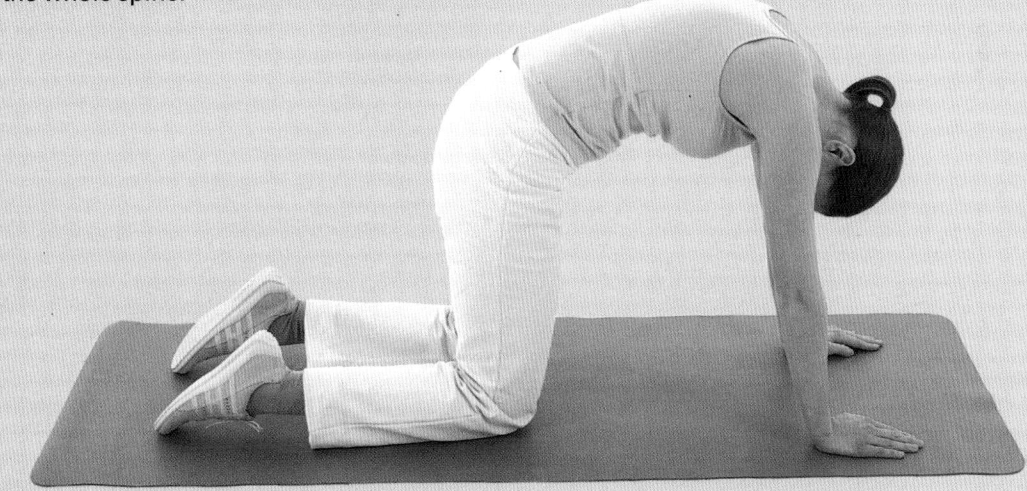

1

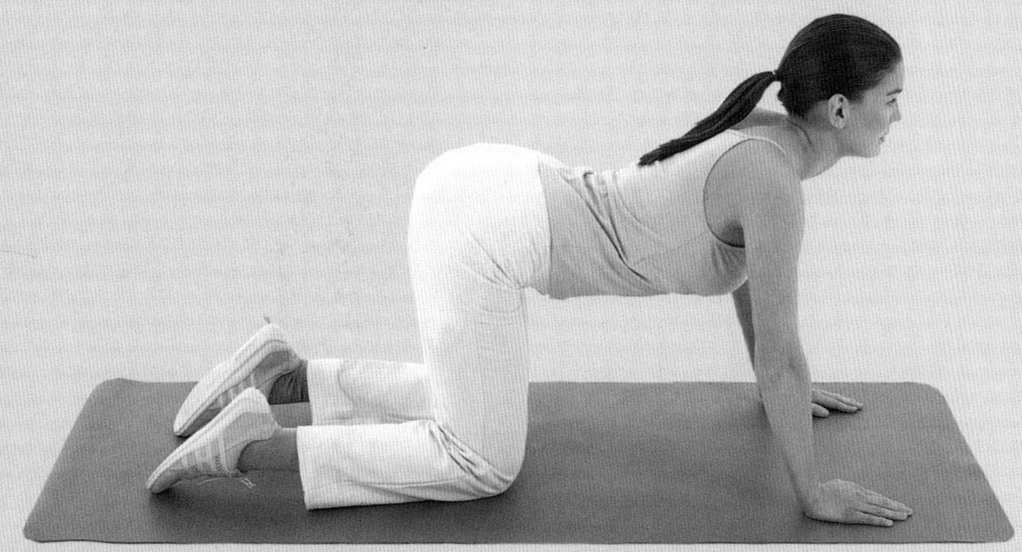

2

Arms and upper body | Week 1

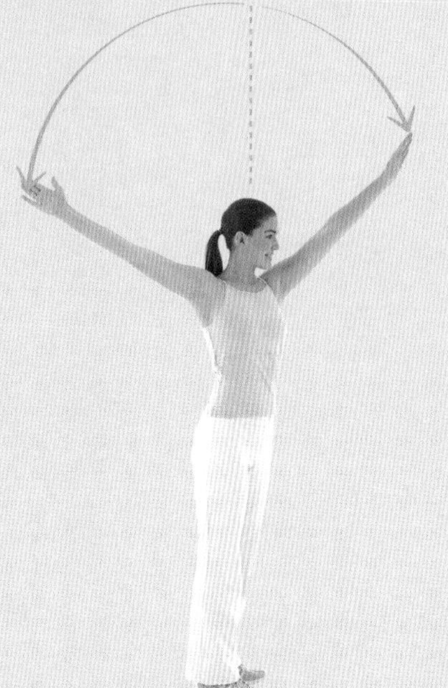

1 Arm jogging

1 Start with both arms above your head. Carefully swing one arm forward and downwards and the other back behind you. Swing both arms in a full circle. If you do the exercise correctly, your arms should cross at the top of the swing above your head.

2 Continue swinging – you may find this takes some concentration! When you have got the arm motion right, try jogging with your legs at the same time. Aim to do 5–10 minutes of this CV exercise.

Focus CV

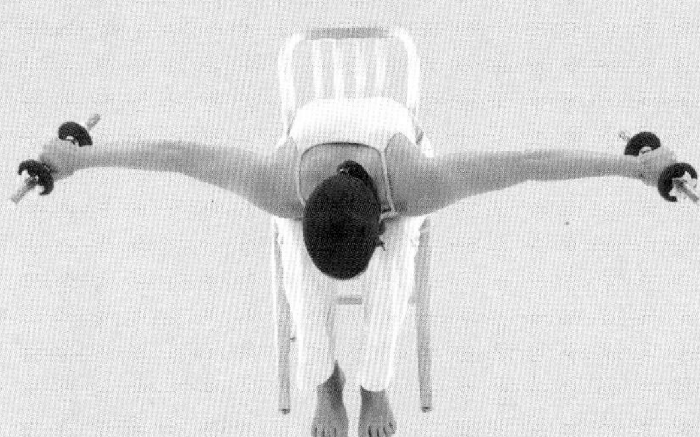

2 One-arm push

1 Assume a Press-up position (see page 99). Move your legs apart to provide some balance and move one arm a little more centrally beneath your body. Now take the other arm off the floor and try to hold the position for 10 seconds. You will feel the weight on your one arm but you must also contract your abdominals and buttocks to help maintain the position. Repeat on the other arm.

Focus Balance

3 Seated-out row

1 Sit on a chair and lean forward to rest on your lap, your head hanging down over your knees and your arms hanging by your sides. Take a dumbbell heavy enough for a '10-rep max' (see page 34) in each hand. Start with your palms facing towards each other and lift both arms out to the side. Lower your arms with control.

Repeat 8 times: raising and lowering your arms counts as 1 move
Focus Toning: rear of shoulder, and upper- and middle-back muscles

4 Syncopated press-up

1 Assume a Press-up position (see top right) and perform a press-up to a six-count move: 1 – lower your body halfway down; 2 – hold; 3 – lower all the way down until your body is just off the floor; 4 – push halfway back up; 5 – hold; 6 – push all the way up.

Repeat this six-count move 4 times. Rest then repeat again
Focus Toning: all the muscles in the arms and chest

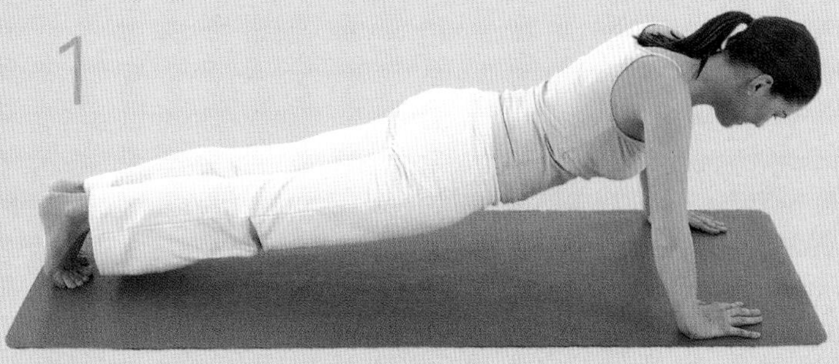

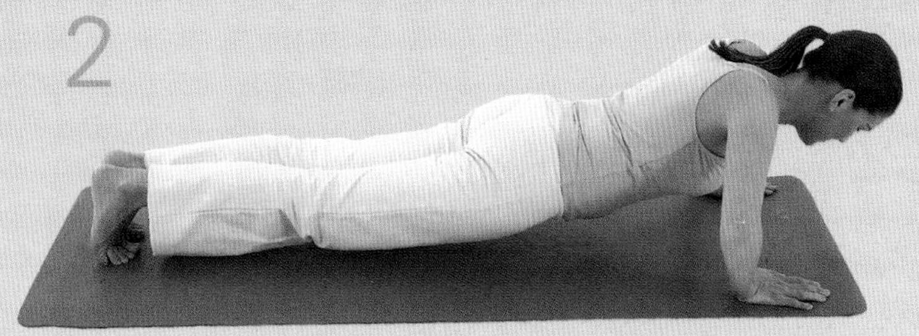

5 Upright row

1 Stand with your feet hip-width apart, your abdominals lifted and both hands holding one dumbbell, which is heavy enough for a '10-rep max' (see page 34).

2 Lift the weight up until it is just beneath your chin, hold, then slowly lower it again. Keep your upper body lifted and not bent over.

Repeat 8 times (or more if your weight isn't heavy enough)
Focus Toning: shoulder and upper back muscles

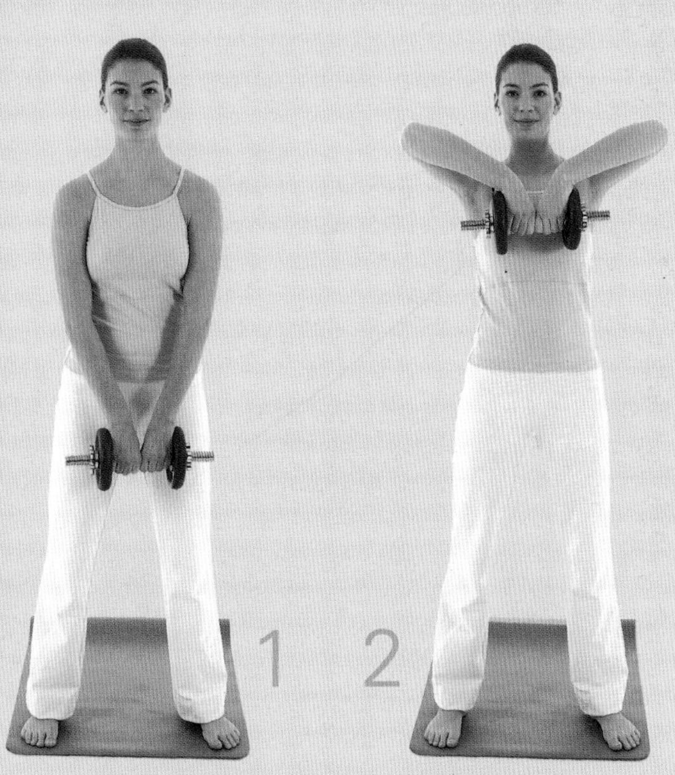

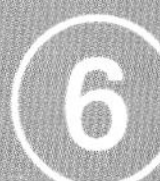

Arms and upper body | Week 2

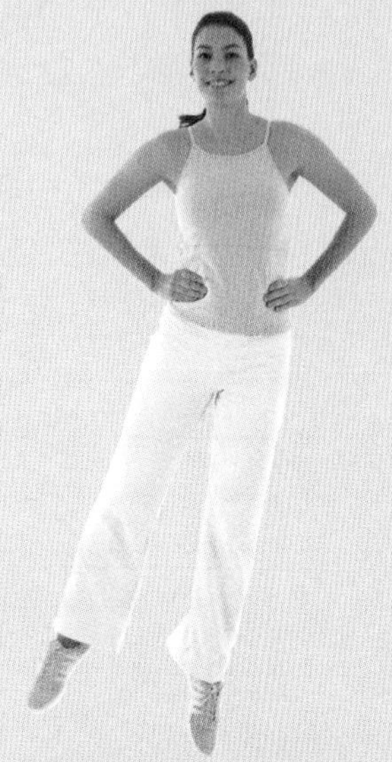

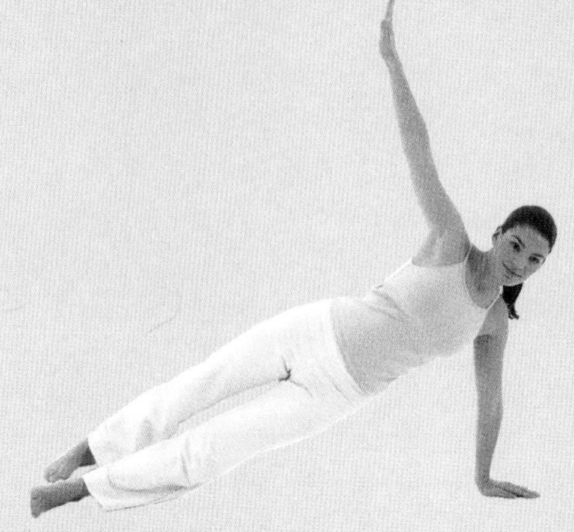

1 Side skipping

1 Gallop to one side, like you did as a child, going round in a circle if you are indoors. Alternate the direction so that each leg is worked equally. After a while add some arm swings in across the body and out to the sides as you skip high and low. Keep going for 10 minutes if you can.

Focus CV

2 Side arch

1 Sit on the floor with your legs outstretched and your hands beside you. Balancing on one arm, lift up your hips, twisting sideways and using your feet to aid your balance. Use your abdominal muscles and raise your upper arm to help you balance. Hold for 15 seconds then lower yourself, using control. Repeat on the other side.

Focus Balance

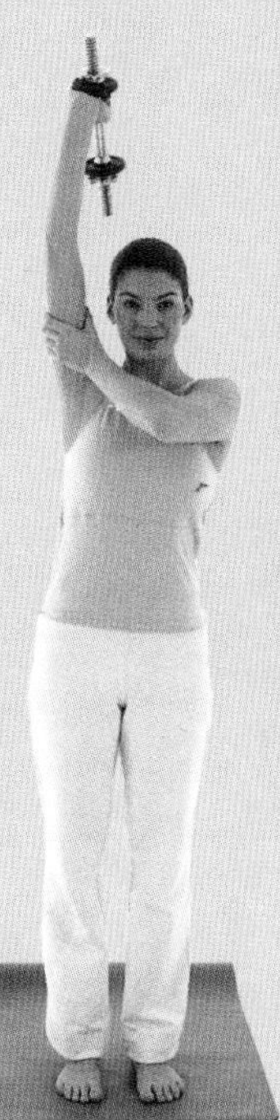

3 Triceps extension

1 Stand with your feet hip-width apart. Take a dumbbell, heavy enough for your '10-rep max' (see page 34) in one hand. Lift the arm toward the ceiling then bend your elbow to drop the arm down behind your shoulder. Support your elbow with the other arm and keep your upper body lifted and upright.

2 Extend the bent arm upwards, pressing the end of the weight toward the ceiling. Keep your abdominals pulled in as you straighten your arm to stop you arching your back. Then slowly lower your arm back down.

Repeat the bend and extention of each arm 8 times
Focus Toning: back of upper arms

▼4 Triceps kickback

1 Hold in one hand the same weight dumbbell as used for the Triceps Extension (opposite) then, leading with the opposite leg, step forward into a lunge. Lean forward with your free hand resting on the forward thigh and lift the elbow of the dumbbell-bearing arm up behind you towards the ceiling.

2 Keeping this elbow and upper arm fixed, extend the lower arm out behind you. Hold this extension then bend the arm in again. Keep the upper arm still as you lift the weight and straighten your arm from the elbow only so as to isolate – and work – the triceps muscle.

Repeat 8 times with each arm
Focus Toning: back of upper arms

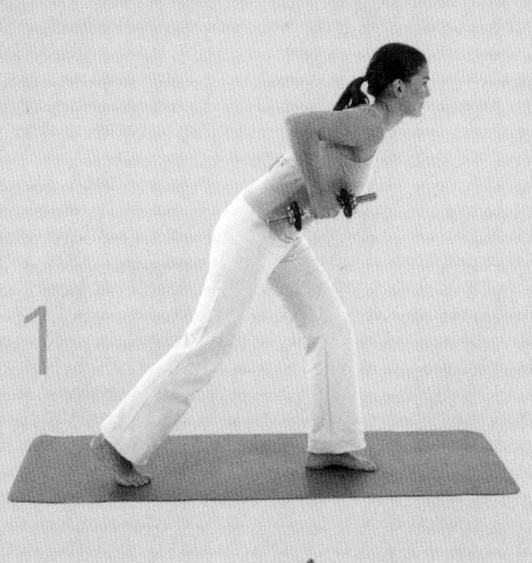
1

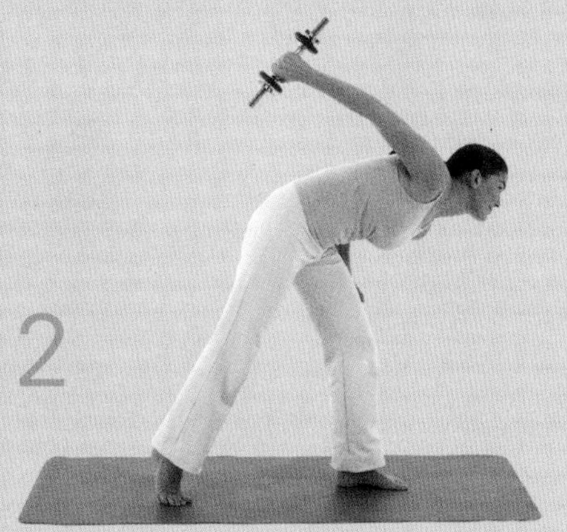
2

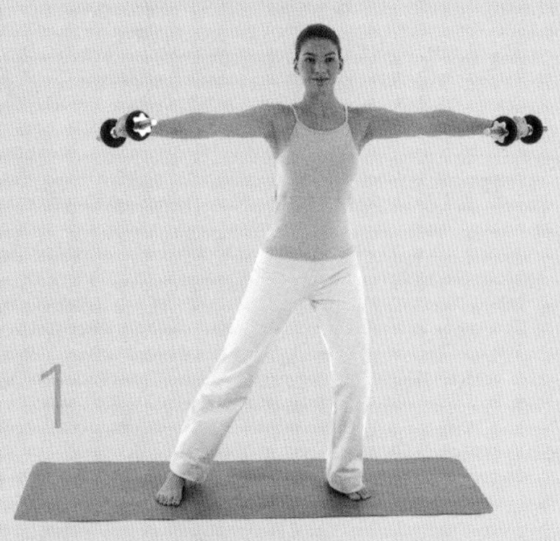
1

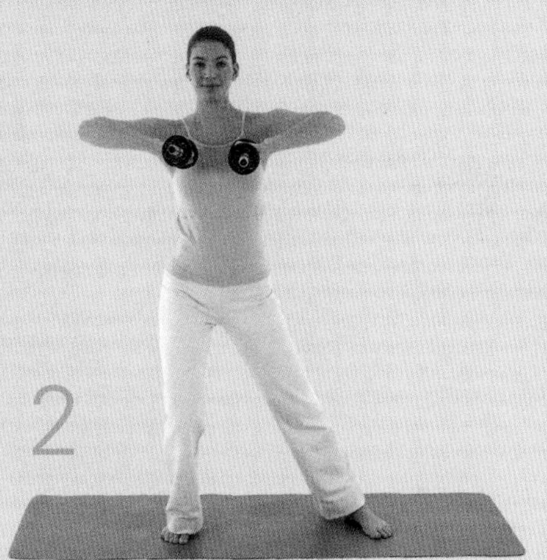
2

▲5 Triceps trick

1 Stand tall with a dumbbell in each hand, your hands meeting in front of your chest. Swing one leg out to the side and step into a lunge position, at the same time opening your arms wide to extend them out to the sides

2 Push off with the foot to return to your starting position and bring both arms back in together as you step in. Keep your abdominals taut as you do this exercise.

Repeat 16 times, moving your arms and legs, then drop your arms to your sides and keep your legs going. When you are ready, resume the arms again
Focus Toning: back of upper arms

Arms and upper body | Week 3

Burpees

1 Start by doing a straight leap into the air, hands above your head. As you land, bend your knees and place your hands on the floor.

2 Jump your feet out behind you into a full Press-up position (see page 99).

3 From here, jump the feet straight back in again and push up into the Upwards Jump. Do 8 to 10 of these moves then jog on the spot to recover your breath before repeating. See if you can keep going in this way for 8 minutes.

Focus CV

3

1

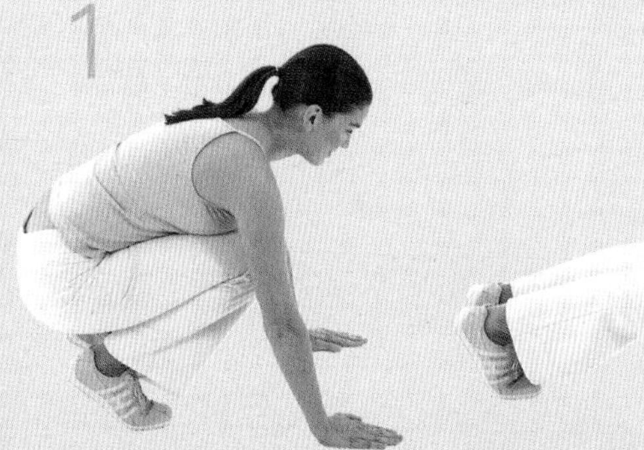

2

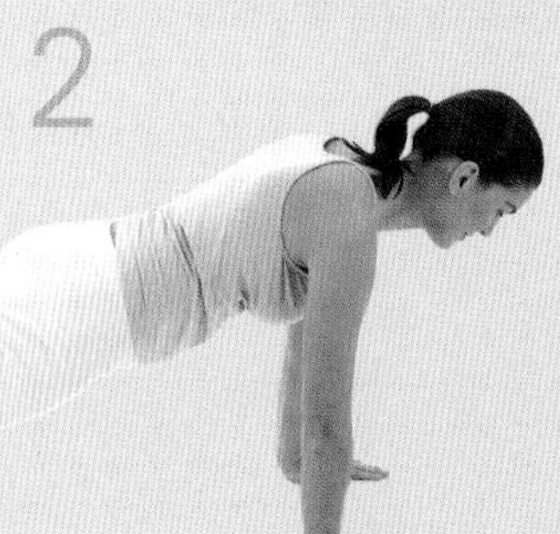

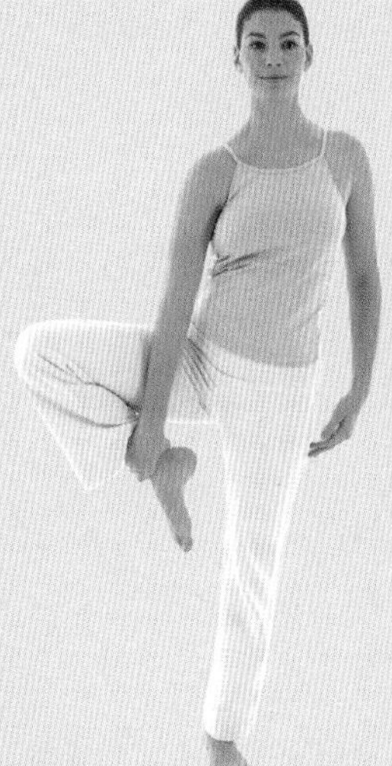

Leg extension

1 Stand on one leg. Take hold of the ankle of the free leg and carefully lift this leg out to the side, keeping the supporting leg as straight as you can. Keep your body lifted too. You may need to put your foot down and try several times to get your balance. Try on each foot – you may find one leg easier to balance on than the other.

Focus Balance

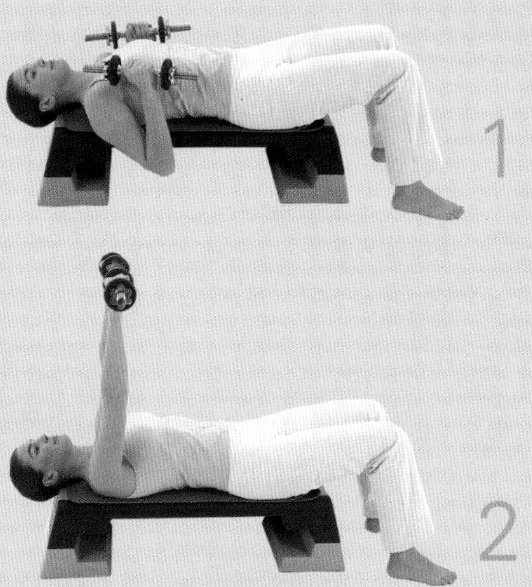

Bench press

1 Lie on your back on a bench with your feet flat on the ground to balance you and a weight in each hand. Start with your elbows bent at right angles and your palms, holding the weights, facing each other.

2 Push your arms straight up toward the ceiling. As you push upwards, turn your palms outwards so that they face your feet when your arms are straight. Bring your arms back down again, turning your palms to face each other once more.

Repeat 8 times or more (depending on the heaviness of the weight)
Focus Toning: chest muscles

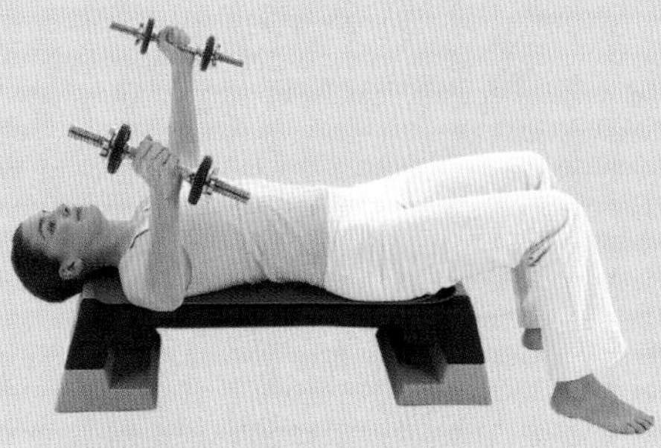

Flat flies

1 Lie on your back on a bench with your feet flat on the ground to balance you. Keeping your elbows slightly bent so as not to lock them, open your arms out wide to the sides with a dumbbell heavy enough for a '10-rep max' (see page 34) in each hand.

2 Bring your arms slowly toward each other until the weights just touch. Slowly open your arms again. Keep your abdominals tight throughout to help maintain your balance.

Repeat 8 times or more (depending on the heaviness of the weight)
Focus Toning: chest muscles

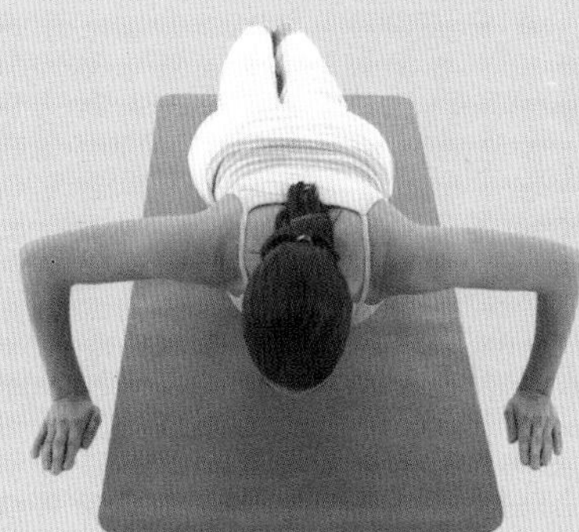

Press-ups

1 Get down on all fours, resting on your hands and knees and keeping your back straight. Place your arms about 1m (3ft) apart and take your legs back behind you so that they are straight, your knees are off the floor and your toes are digging into the floor.

2 Using your arms, lower your body until your chest is just off the floor, then push back to an upright position.

Repeat press-up 10 times, rest, then repeat again
Focus Toning: arm and chest muscles

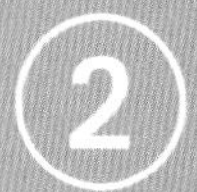

Arms and upper body | **Week 4**

1 Sky jumping

1 From a standing position, bend down and touch the floor, then touch your knees, then jump and reach for the sky.

2 Do at least 8 to 10 of these jumps then, when you get too out of breath or your legs ache too much to continue, do some On-the-Spot Jogging or jogging around the room to recover. Keep alternating the Sky Jumps with jogging for 20 minutes.

Focus CV

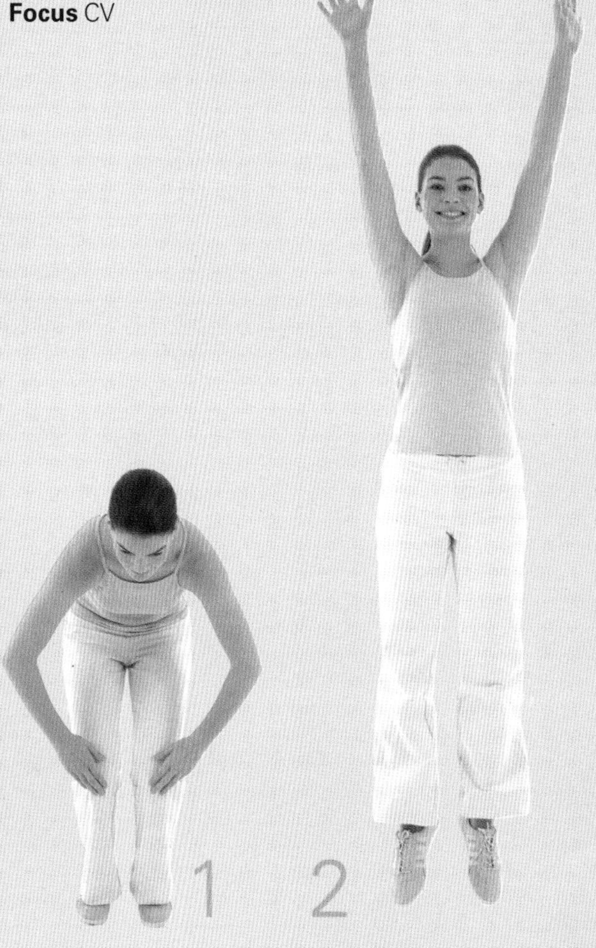

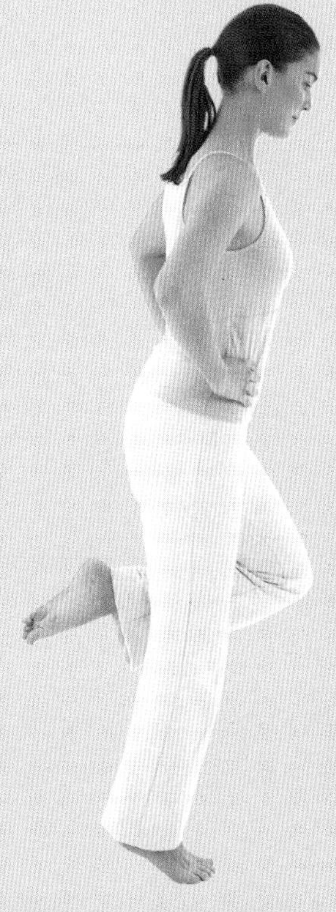

2 Leg-heel raise

1 Stand with your feet hip-width apart and lift up your heels until you are on tiptoe, pulling up on your abdominals to help you balance. Hold this position then lift one foot just off the floor and try to continue the balance. It will become easier the more you practise. Repeat the balance on the other leg.

Focus Balance

3 Shoulder press

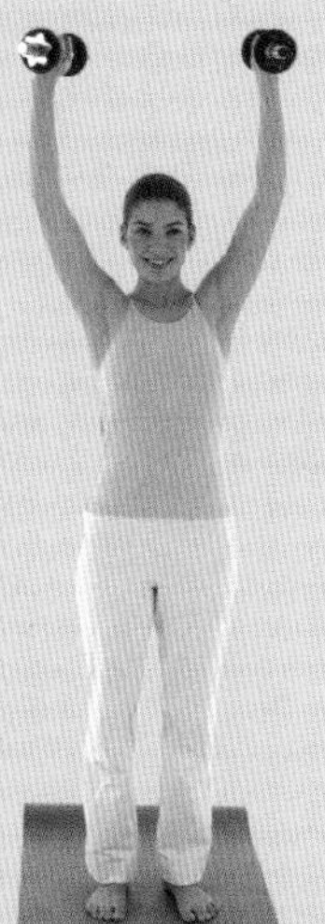

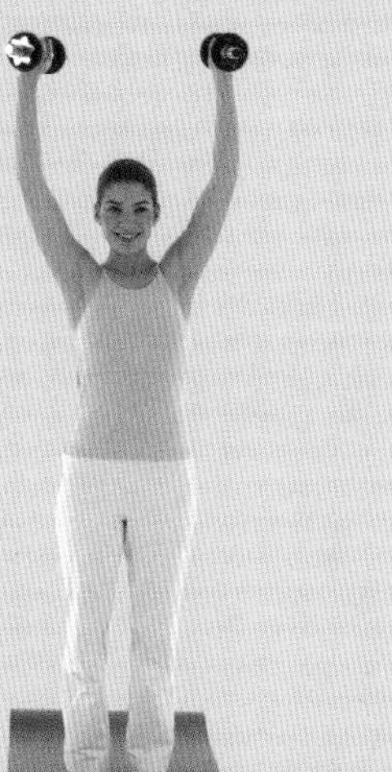

1 Stand tall with your legs hip-width apart and a dumbbell, heavy enough for your '10-rep max' (see page 34), in each hand. Hold the weights near your shoulders. Keep your abdominals pulled in and push both arms straight up toward the ceiling, then lower carefully. Take care that you don't allow your back to arch as you tire.

Repeat 8 times
Focus Toning: shoulder muscles

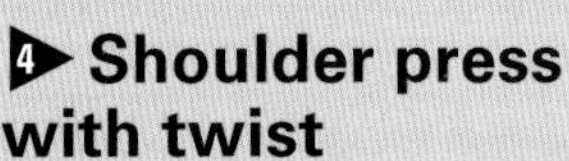

4 Shoulder press with twist

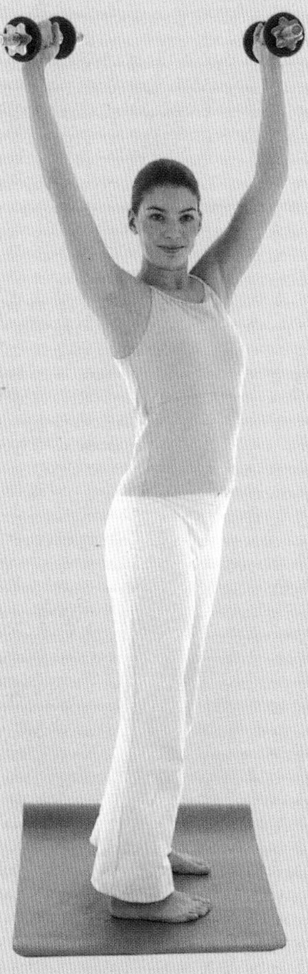

1 Do the same Shoulder Press as above but as you lift your arms towards the ceiling, twist your upper body a quarter turn to face the side. As you twist you are overloading one shoulder muscle more than the other. Twist back as you carefully lower your arms.

Repeat 8 times with a twist on each side
Focus Toning: shoulder muscles

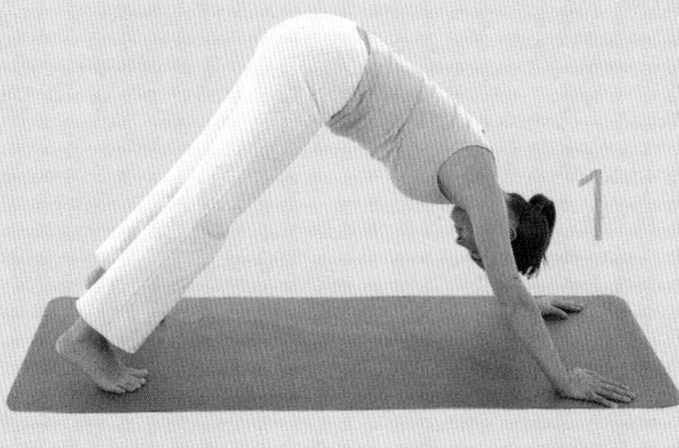
1

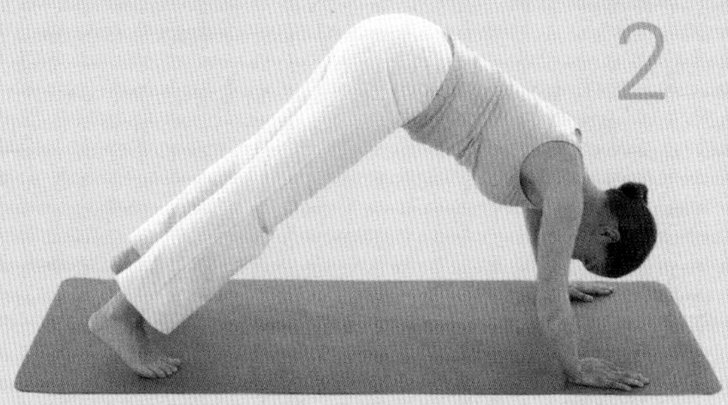
2

5 Tiger press-up

1 Assume a Press-up position (see page 99), but then suck in your abdominals and lift your hips towards the ceiling so that you are in an upside-down V-shape.

2 Now try to bend your arms and lower your head toward the floor. Press your arms straight to lift up again. Lowering and raising the body in this way, as opposed to the normal press-up position, puts the focus of this exercise on the shoulders.

Repeat 10 times
Focus Toning: shoulder muscles

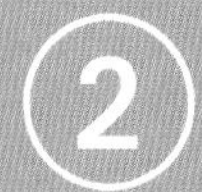

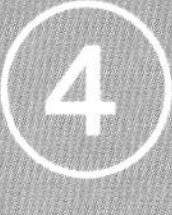

Arms and upper body | Week 5

1 CV combination 1

Make up a routine that lasts at least 25 minutes by combining all of the following:

- Arm Jogging (see page 98)
- Side Skipping (see page 100)
- Burpees (see page 102)
- Sky Jumping (see page 104)

Breathe steadily throughout and if the exercise feels too tough, slow it down a little until you get your breath back.

Focus CV

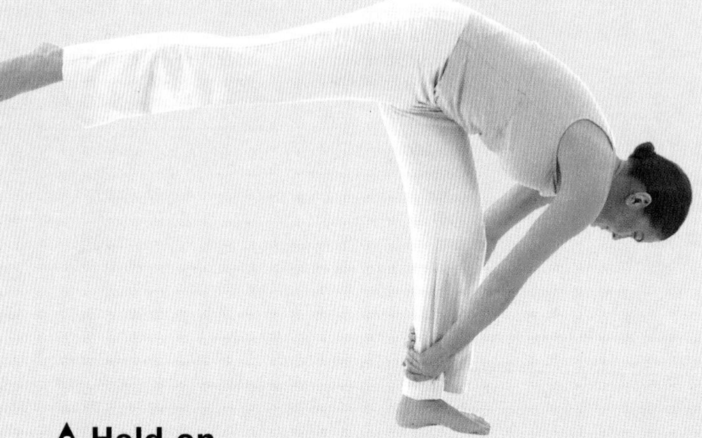

2 Hold-on

1 From a standing position, bend over and take hold of one ankle with both hands. Now lift and stretch the free leg up behind you as far as you can, holding on to your abdominals to hold the balance. Aim to get the leg straight, if possible, with your head toward the knee of the supporting leg. Repeat on the other leg. If you find it too hard to balance, rest one hand on the floor to support yourself.

Focus Balance

3 Shadow boxing 1

1 Skipping lightly from one foot to the other, punch your arms forward as if in a boxing match. Throw a punch – jabbing the fist forwards in an aggressive manner and then drawing the arm back in again. Try doing multiple jabs with one fist then the other. Now try alternating jabs or pretending you have a punch bag in front of you.

Repeat the skipping and jabbing movements for a full 5 minutes
Focus Toning: upper arms, shoulder and upper- and middle-back muscles

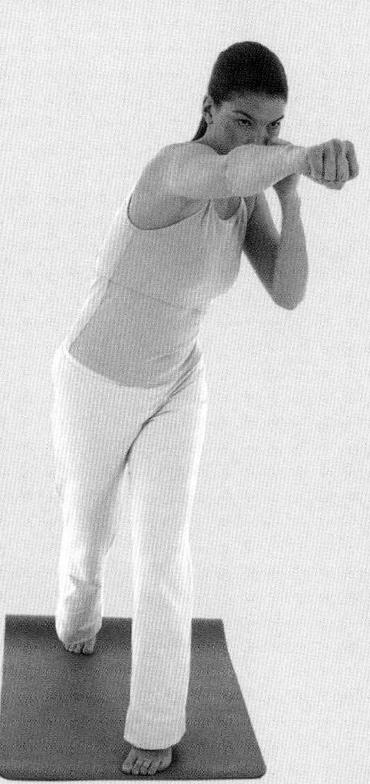

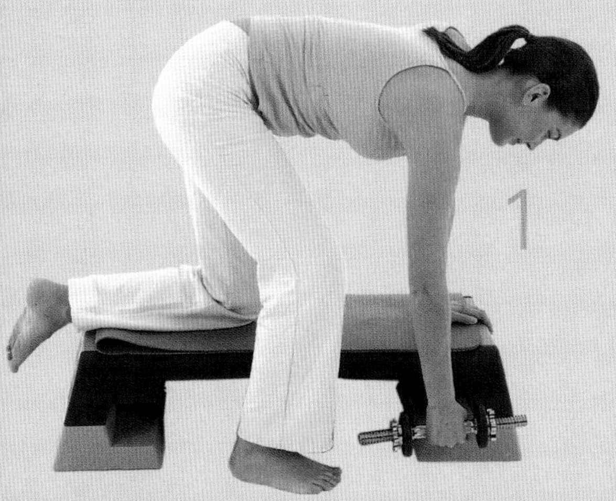

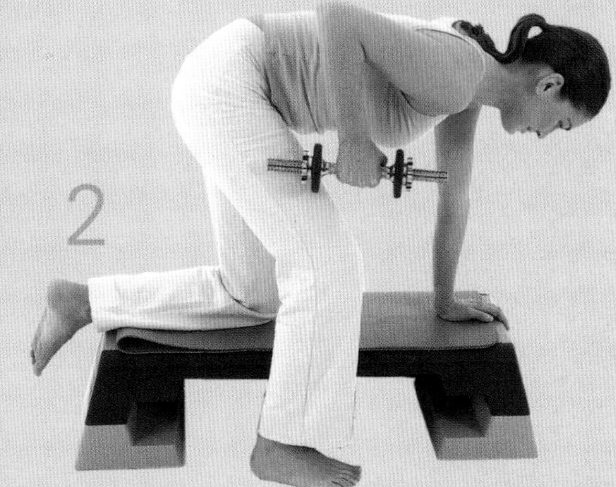

4 Single-arm row

1 Rest one knee on a bench or couch. Let the arm on the opposite side hang down, holding in your hand a dumbbell heavy enough for a '10-rep max' (see page 34). Support your body weight on the other arm.

2 Lift the weight toward your chest raising your elbow toward the ceiling, hold then lower again.

Repeat lifts 8 times on each arm
Focus Toning: upper arms and shoulder muscles

5 Prone lift

1 Lie flat on your front with your arms out to the side, palms facing the floor. Now lift both arms upwards slightly then lower them again. Keep breathing and keep your abdominals tight.

Repeat lifts 15 times, rest, then repeat
Focus Toning: muscles between the shoulder blades

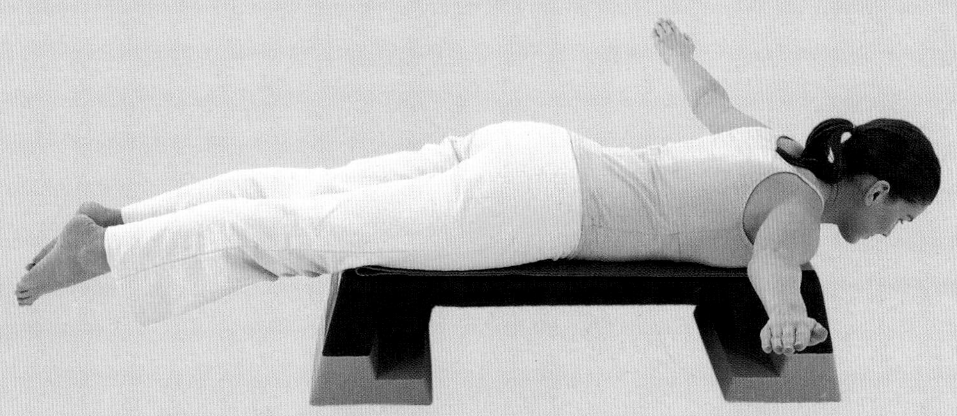

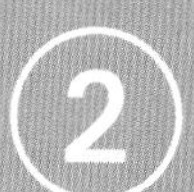

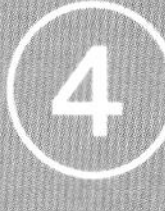

6

Arms and upper body | Week 6

1 CV combination 2

Make up a routine that lasts up to 30 minutes by combining all of the following:

- Arm Jogging (see page 98)
- Side Skipping (see page 100)
- Burpees (see page 102)
- Sky Jumping (see page 104)

To increase the intensity and really get your heart pumping, jog on the spot in between each exercise for 1 minute.

Focus CV

2 Handstand

1 From a standing position, place your hands on the floor, tuck your head between your hands and with one leg kick off the floor and up into a handstand, resting your upturned feet against a wall if necessary. With all the toning work you have been doing you should be able to hold your balance for some seconds then bring one leg down slowly to come back to an upright position.

Focus Balance

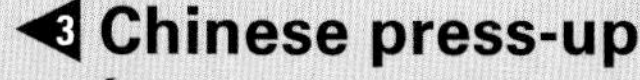

3 Chinese press-up

1 Assume the Press-up position (see page 99) but place your hands just shoulder-width apart and keep your elbows into your sides, not out at right angles, as usual. As you lower into the Press-up, keep your elbows touching the sides of your ribcage so as to work your triceps muscles. Press upwards in the same way.

Repeat Press-ups 20 times
Focus Toning: back of upper arms

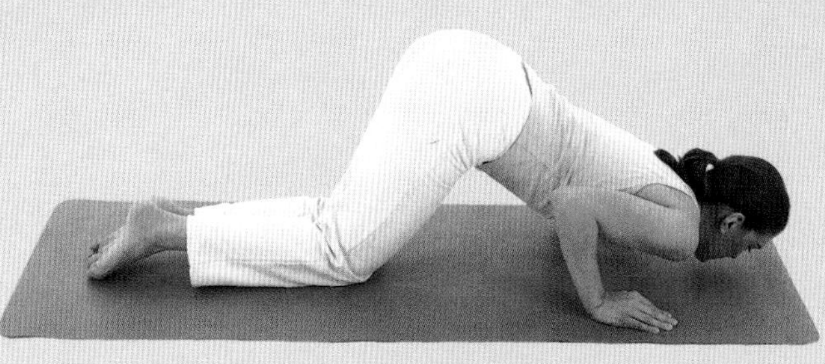

4 Cheating row

1 Adopt the position of the Single-Arm Row (see page 107), taking a weight in one hand as before.

2 Lift your arm in the same way, but this time as you lift, twist your upper body in the direction you are pulling the arm. Lower your arm back down and allow your upper body to twist back to face the floor again.

Repeat lifts 8 times on each arm
Focus Toning: upper ribcage and side abdominal muscles, plus upper arm muscles

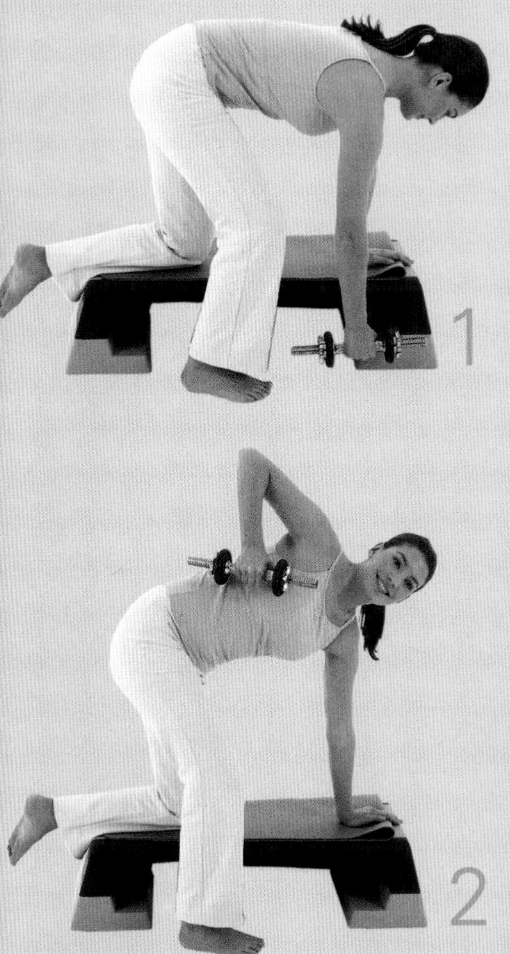

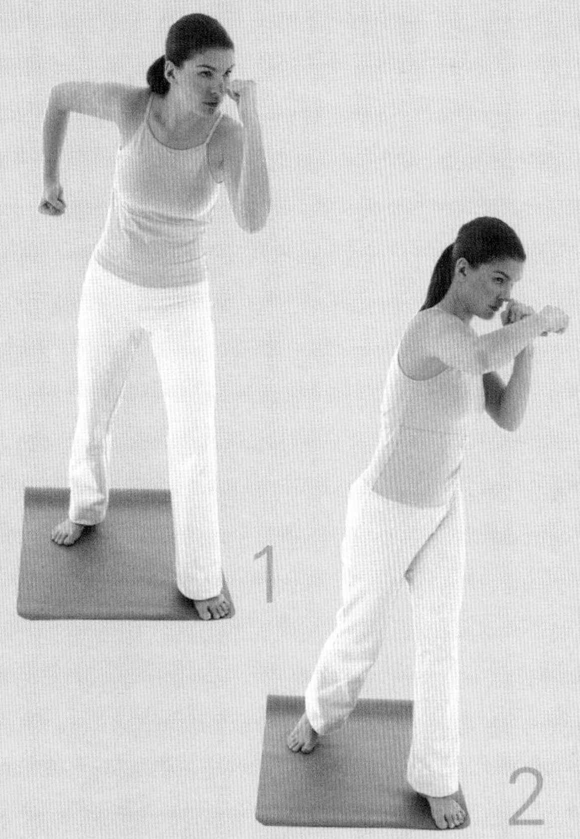

5 Shadow boxing 2

1 Skip on the spot, throwing jabs at an imaginary opponent, as you did for Shadow Boxing 1 (see page 106), but this time add some upper-cut punches. Using your whole body, swing your arm upwards with force from low down, bringing your fist up as though hitting someone beneath the chin. Alternate these punches with the jabs and keep switching arms to exercise them equally. You should feel breathless after this exercise as you are using more than just the arm muscles as you punch and skip on the spot.

Repeat the jabs for 2 minutes on each arm or make up your own sequence of punches
Focus Toning: upper arms, shoulder and chest muscles

ARMS AND UPPER BODY

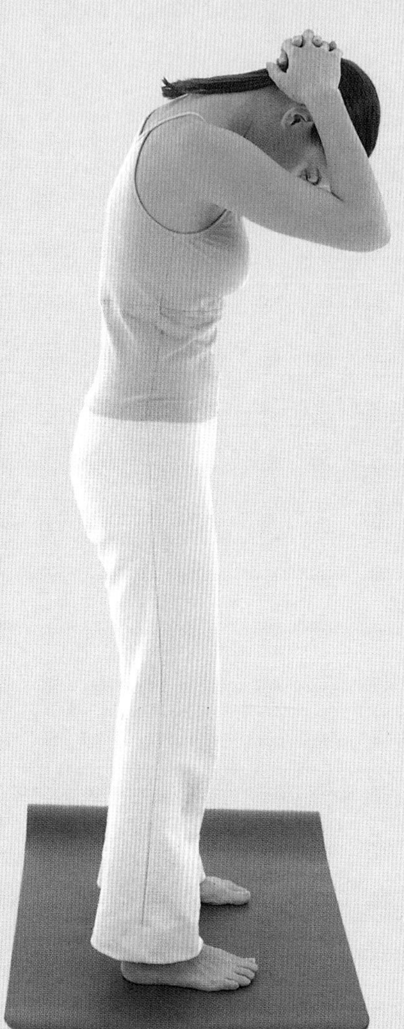

2 Open the bridge

1 Stand with your feet wide apart and clasp your hands together behind your back. Lean your upper body over toward the floor, bring your hands over the top of your upturned head and press them as far forward as you can. Hold for 10–15 seconds, then lift your arms to bring you back to an upright position. Repeat again.

1 Neck stretch

1 Stand with your hands clasped behind your head and bow your head forward. Keep your upper body lifted, keep your abdominals tight and only let the head come forwards. Use the weight of your hands to pull down on the head, further stretching the muscles at the base of the neck. Hold for 10–15 seconds then release.

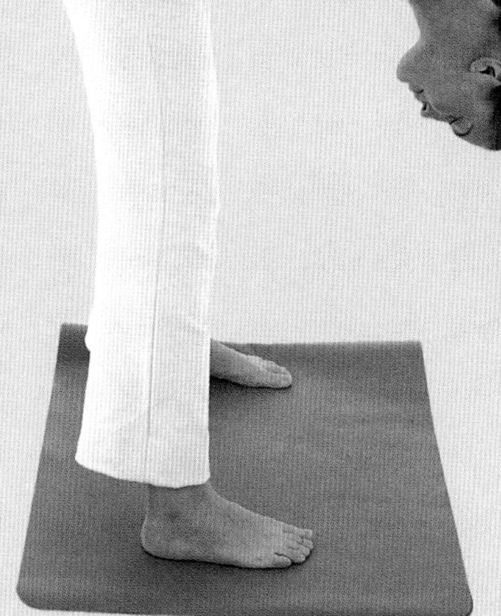

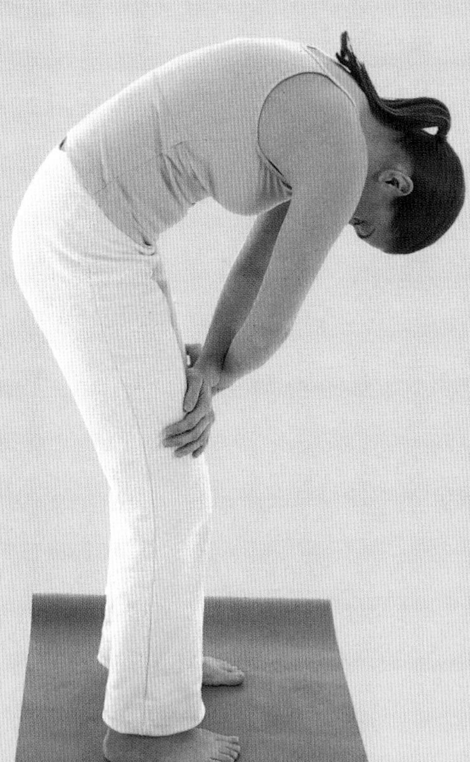

3 Upper body fold

1 From a standing position stick your bottom out behind you and bend your knees so that you are in a squat position. Cross your arms and place your hands on opposite knees. Now suck your navel toward your spine and round your back, pushing it out as far as you can. You will feel this gentle stretch in the middle upper back – and possibly even in the lower back. Hold for a few seconds while breathing normally then release to a straight back. Repeat the arch three more times.

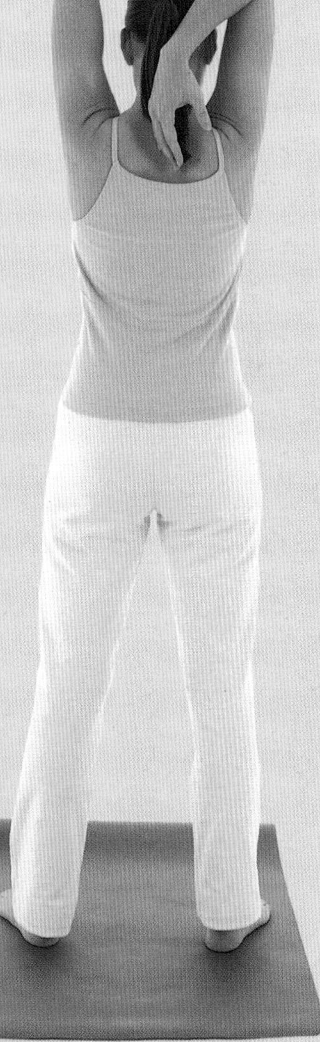

4 Triceps stretch

1 Stand squarely and place your right hand back over your right shoulder. Lift your right elbow up towards the ceiling. Use your left arm to help press the elbow back further. Tense your abdominals to keep from tipping back too far. Hold for 10–15 seconds then do the same on the left arm.

Building your own programme

You should now have worked your way through one of the six-week programmes and got a taste for hard work. You will notice that the exercises become progressively more challenging over the weeks; however, if you need to challenge yourself further you can always increase the number of repetitions you do. Better still, you can increase the number of times you work through the whole week's routine. You should be aiming to do the workout outlined for each week at least three times during that week. If you can fit in four times, even better!

Make the best of your time

Give the moves the concentration they deserve and stay mindful of your technique throughout your workout. You should always try to stand tall with your abdominals lifted and tightened to support the torso.

Aim to train at the same time each week or put aside a time for your routine when you know you will not be interrupted. Once you start your routine, aim to finish it – don't allow yourself to become distracted by the telephone or television.

The cardiovascular (CV) work suggested is important so try to fit this in each time. CV work is aerobic and uses up stored fat as energy and will reduce your fat stores so that your true shape starts to come through.

Seeing results

Once you get training on one area you will notice how your muscles are shaping up and becoming more defined. Take another look at yourself in the mirror after six weeks and reassess. Now you can start to see your body's shape more you can decide on your next routine. You may have lost some body fat, for example, and decide that your hips need flattening down a little. Whatever you decide, you will have valuable information about which body areas to work on next. Remember this programme is flexible, so mix and match the different workouts to suit your goals. If you keep changing your routine every six weeks, you will stay challenged and motivated!

Ideas for your next programme

- **If you have a thick waist, do the arms and upper body programme to build up the shoulders. This will even out your shape and make your waist seem thinner**
- **If you are concerned about your heavy thighs, do the legs and thighs programme**
- **If you feel bottom heavy, do the bottom and hips programme followed by the legs and thighs programme**
- **If you have worked on the stomach area already but are still not satisfied, repeat the six-week abdominal shaping programme placing extra emphasis on the CV part**
- **If you want to mix and match for a change, take an exercise from each body part and build your weeks that way**

Keeping up the good work

Keeping up a fitness programme is hard work and there may be times when you lack enthusiasm. This book is designed to make motivation easier because, with its six-week programmes, you are working towards a reachable goal each time.

When you complete a six-week stint, take a look in the mirror and congratulate yourself. Six weeks of consistent work will have benefited you inside and out. Give yourself a treat to reward yourself.

Don't worry if at the end of six weeks you don't feel like going straight back into another programme and on to another body part. Try a different activity for a few weeks instead – the important thing is that you keep some form of exercise going on a regular basis to maintain your new shape and improved muscle tone. Keep the book handy – then whenever you feel your body needs a quick intense boost, start a six-week programme and make sure you finish it!

Motivational tips

- If you don't feel like doing your workout one day – try to ignore the feeling and at least start the routine. Once you have done even 5 minutes of exercise you will be surprised at how much better you feel and you may well go on to finish the whole routine. Afterwards you will feel so glad you did it
- Don't let tiredness stop you. Even though you may feel you cannot walk another step, a gentle exercise session will leave you with more energy than when you started. As you continue your sessions you will build more muscles and you will start to notice small changes. Perhaps you feel less tired, or perhaps your posture is improving. These things will inspire you towards greater effort
- Don't use the excuse of 'I haven't got time'. If you don't have the time, do 5 minutes anyway. If you regularly exercise your heart, you will find running for the bus will not leave you exhausted for the whole morning, and with blood flowing more efficiently you will get through your tasks quicker, leaving you with more time and more energy
- If you are feeling really unmotivated treat yourself to a new pair of trainers or a new set of training pants. You will be surprised at what a new lease of life some new gear can give you
- If you have skipped a session, don't give up. These things happen so battle on towards your six-week goal and you will get there
- If you are bored with the routine, the great thing about the layout of this book is that it allows you to mix and match a little. Swap programmes for a few days or choose your favourite exercises. Just do the stretches if you want or focus on the CV exercises
- Take a picture of yourself before you start your programme – this will inspire you to keep working toward your goal

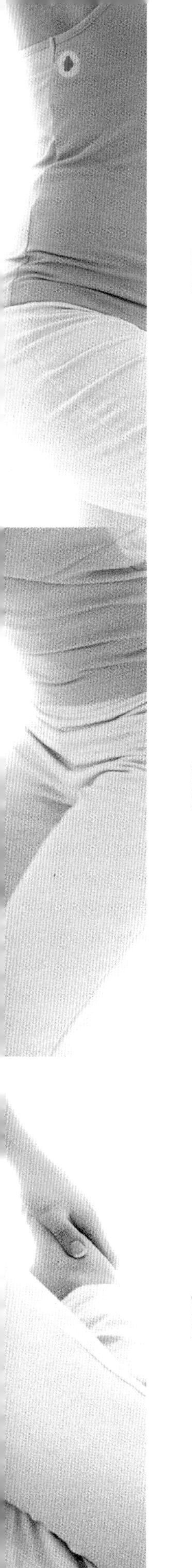

post-natal exercises

bad backs

increased flexibility

corrective shaping

Shaping up for life

Now that you have learned how to use this book – keep it handy. Use it as a reference book for when there is a specific part of your body with which you feel unhappy. If you want to do a more overall programme then you can always take exercises from different areas of the book to make up a more varied routine. Alternatively, there may be times when you get involved in other sports or activities but feel that you need a few exercises to tone up a certain part of your body that may be overlooked in your chosen sport. This is when you can take this book down from the bookshelf and refer to it again.

General wellbeing

Body sculpting, or corrective shaping, is really about strengthening the areas that need it, while keeping flexible at the same time. This is important for your body shape and look, but it is also important for your health. You may well have approached your workouts from the viewpoint of your end appearance. You will have realized, however, that as you improve the look and shape of your body, you are also improving its strength and alignment, thereby allowing it to function better, too.

There may be times when you feel you need some corrective work on your body that is less to do with shape and more to do with overall wellbeing. After a specific 'trauma', such as pregnancy, the body needs extra help in rejuvenating itself. The body of a woman who has been through nine months of pregnancy and then several months of caring for a tiny baby, with all the associated reduced sleep and increased demands on her time, could well use some corrective shaping. If this applies to you, the gentle corrective type of exercises on pages 118–121 will help you strengthen and mobilize the parts of your body that most need it and help you on your way to full body recovery.

Also included in this chapter are corrective exercises for the back – one of the most common areas prone to injury. The exercises on page 122–123 will strengthen the erector spinae muscles that run along the length of the spine. Strengthening these muscles and the other muscles around the torso area will help protect your back.

Finally, this chapter focuses on developing stretching to increase flexibility. As we get older our mobility can become reduced which, if we become too sedentary, can lead to our bodies becoming stiffer. On pages 124–125 you will find some further stretches that help loosen the muscles and ligaments and promote flexibility. These types of stretches should be done regularly to extend, elongate and keep the mobility in all areas of the body.

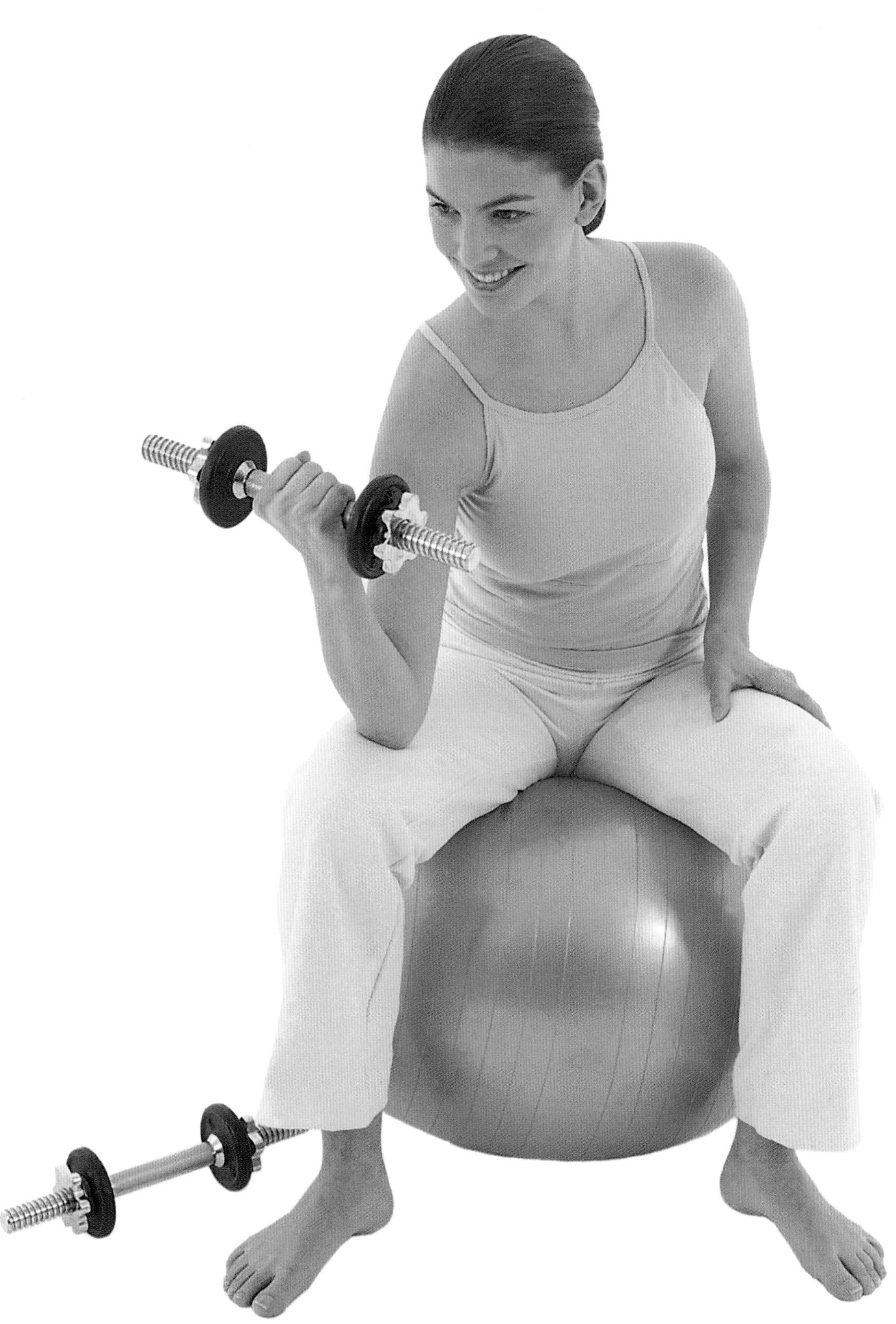

POST-NATAL EXERCISES

The two key areas that need work when you have just had a baby are the stomach and the back. Your abdominal muscles will have been stretched out of shape during the nine months of the baby's development inside. At the same time, the back is forced into an exaggerated bend and takes extra weight. In addition, the back becomes less stable as the relaxin hormone kicks in and softens the mother's ligaments. Therefore any post-natal programme needs to focus on strengthening the whole torso area as effectively as possible.

Try the following exercises to take your first steps towards post-natal strengthening and body sculpting:

1 Pelvic tilt

If you had a normal delivery, these exercises can be done after your six-week check-up. If you had a Caesarean section you should wait 12 weeks before starting.

2 Head lift

As you start to become stronger you can start adding in this exercise, which follows on from the Pelvic Tilt above and further engages your abdominal muscles.

3 Full-flat curl

This final phase of abdominal rehabilitation will build you back up to doing a normal Curl-up move.

1 Pelvic tilt

1 Lie on your back with your knees bent, your feet flat on the floor and your arms relaxed by your sides. Lie for a moment and just feel the floor beneath you.

2 Now think about the stomach muscles lying across the top of your abdomen area and start to contract them. As you do this, aim to push your lower back in toward the floor. Hold the position for a moment then release your back to its original position. This is a basic pelvic tilt and it re-establishes the working relationship between your stomach muscles and your back.

3 Perform 8 of these tilts, resting as often as you need to if your stomach muscles feel tired.

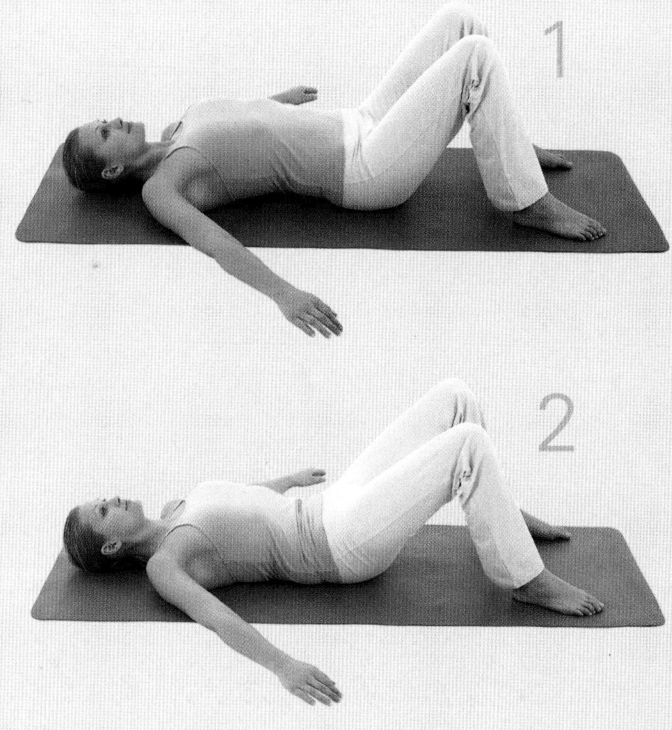

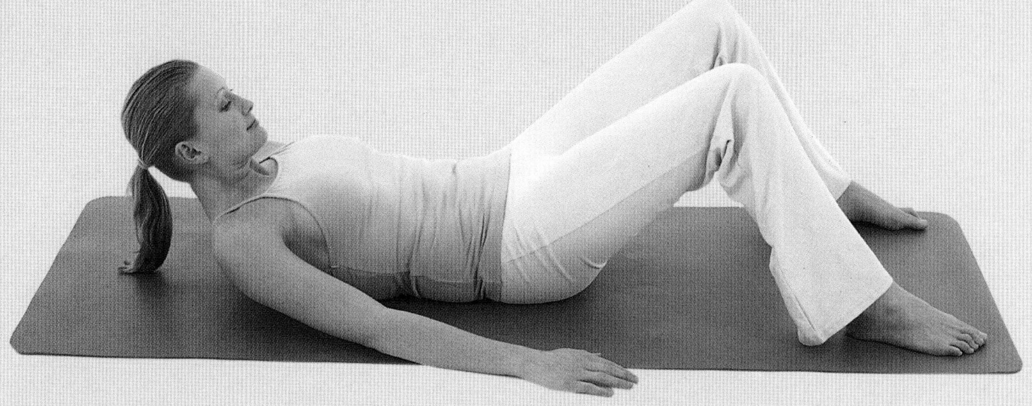

▲2 Head lift

1 Lie on your back as before but this time, after you have performed the pelvic tilt, start to lift your head slowly off the floor, leaving your hands by your sides. Lift only until you can feel your abdominals contracting, then slowly lower your head back down again.

2 Do 8 to 10 of these lifts and you will recontact the abdominal muscles as well as working the neck muscles a little.

▼3 Full-flat curl

1 Lie on your back as before, but place your hands beneath your head. Lift your head and shoulders off the floor but keep staring at your stomach instead of lifting your chin away from your chest as you would do in a normal Curl-up. By gazing at your stomach area you keep it as flat as possible as you lift and lower your head.

2 Aim to perform 8 to 10 of these Curl-ups slowly.

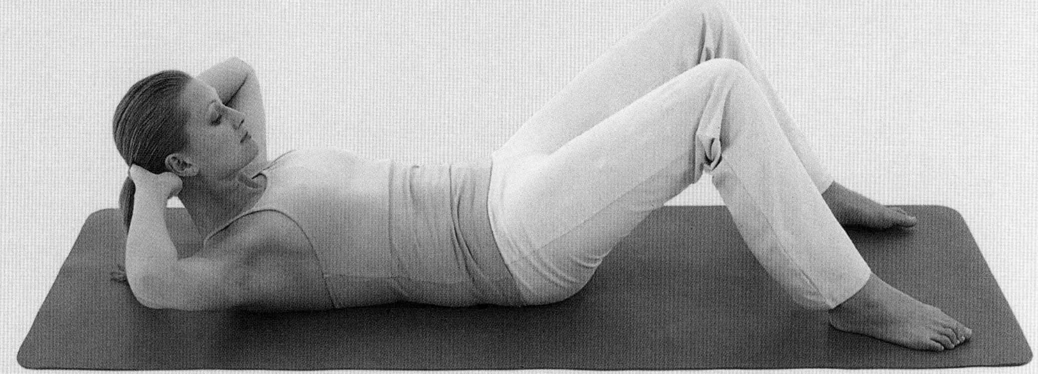

POST-NATAL EXERCISES CONTINUED

As your baby grows and your body recovers you can begin to extend the range of exercises you are doing. From the sixth week of exercising onwards, for example, you can start to include some more cardiovascular movements and also some more work for the back.

Start your mini-workout with the Stepping 1 exercise on page 78. The stepping movements can be built up gradually and will get your heart, lungs and your muscles working. Then do the following exercises.

4 Cat arch

This movement flexes and mobilizes the back.

5 Hyperextension 1

Caution: this exercise may not be comfortable for breast-feeding mums and therefore should be avoided if it causes any pain to the breasts.

4 Cat arch

1 Get down on all fours, resting on your hands and knees and draw in your stomach as much as you can – really feel like you are pulling your navel toward the back of your spine. As you do this, allow your back to arch upwards like a cat.

2 Hold this position for a moment then slowly release your back and return to your original position. Do 10–12 of these arches slowly and carefully.

1

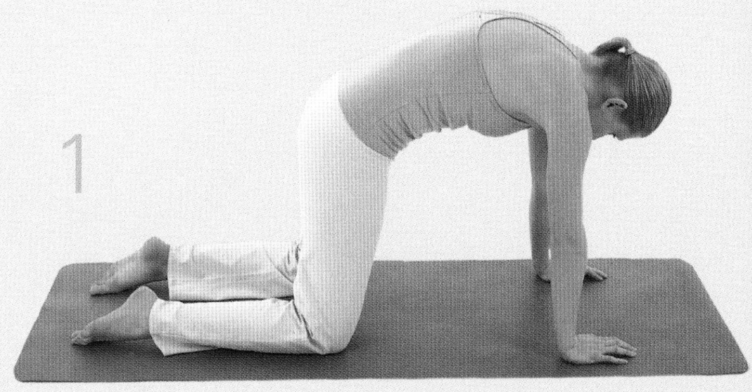

2

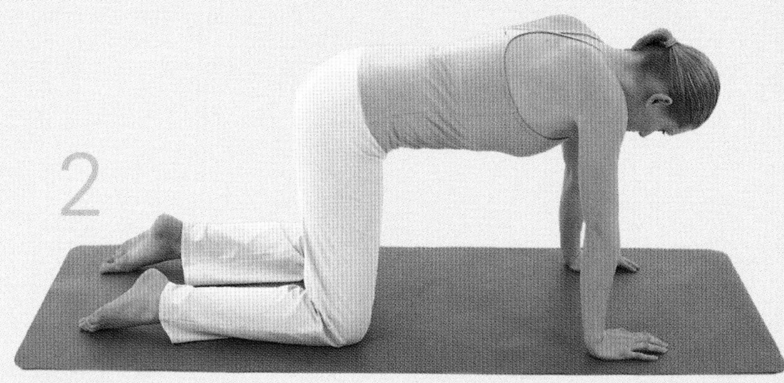

5 Hyperextension 1

1 Lie flat on your front with your arms back and your hands clasped behind you. Contract your buttock muscles and try to lift your head and shoulders off the floor, leaving your hands on the floor. Repeat 4 times, then lower and rest.

2 Now place your hands on your shoulders and do 8 full lifts. Slowly lower yourself down to the ground and rest.

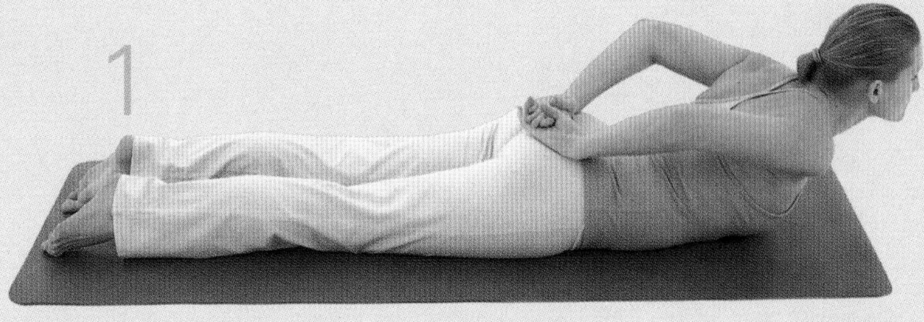

1

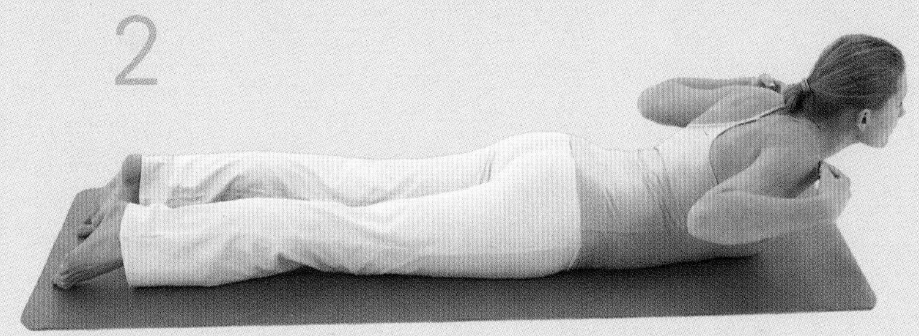

2

6 Squat

Practise the Squat 1 exercise on page 79 as much as you can throughout your day, for example when you bend to lift your baby off the floor, when you reach down to change a nappy or you stand over the cot looking in. Even do 5 or 6 of these after you have been to the toilet. If you use the squat move every time you bend you will protect your back and strengthen and tone your legs and bottom in the process.

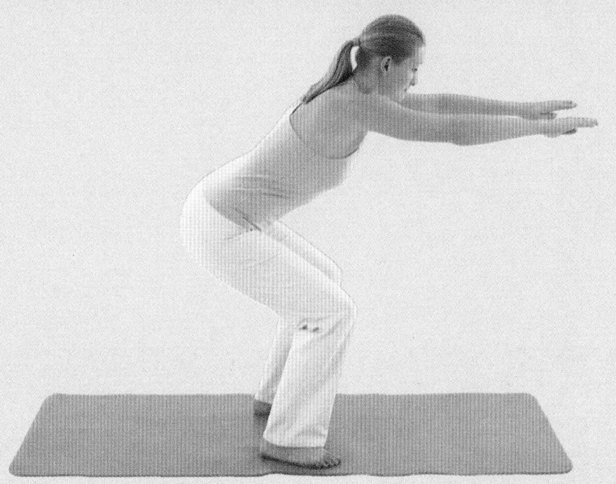

Additional exercises

As the weeks go by, add in some other exercises from the six-week body-sculpting programmes to your routine, in particular:

- Week 1, Stomach and Waist (see page 42)
- Week 2, Legs and Thighs (see page 80)
- Week 1, Arms and Upper Body (see page 98)

When you feel really ready for a challenge try the six-week Stomach and Waist programme, which begins on page 40, and build up your exercise from there.

BAD BACKS

Corrective exercise can also be used for problem areas prone to injury, one of the most common of which is the back. This is often as a result of mistreatment of the back – we load heavy weights on to our torsos and twist and push our spines into positions they are not really designed for. In addition, we often fail to strengthen the muscles needed to keep our backs in good condition.

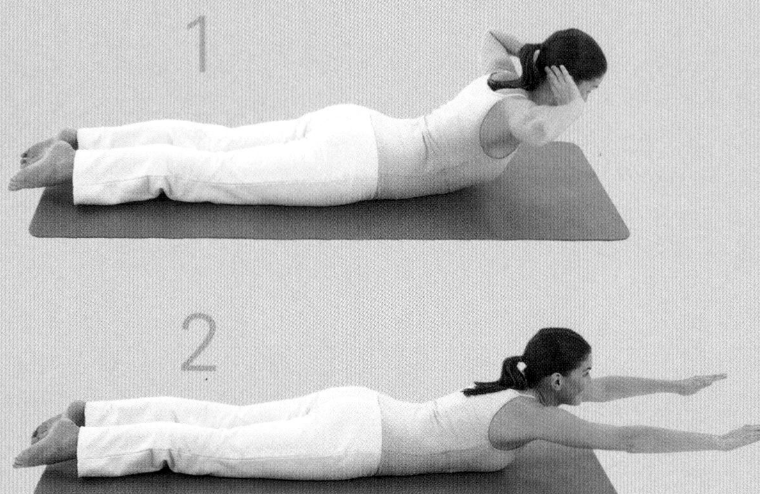

Corrective treatment for backs

Start, if necessary, by losing some weight. The quickest way to shift excess body fat is with cardiovascular (CV) exercise. Use any or all of the CV exercises in this book to build yourself some daily programmes of 20–30 minutes. Note, if your back is particularly bad you may need to avoid the high-impact exercises, such as jumping, in the book.

The next step is to strengthen the erector spinae muscles, which run along the length of the spine. Perform the exercises on these two pages as well as the following:

- Tension Hold 1 (see page 44)
- Lower Abs 1 (see page 47)
- Yoga Arch and Shoot-Outs (see page 50)

⚠1 Hyperextension 2

1 Lie flat on your front with your elbows bent and your hands behind your head. As you contract your buttock muscles and lift your head and shoulders off the floor you have the extra weight of your hands to lift which makes it harder work for the back muscles. Lift as high as you can then lower again slowly.

2 To make this even more challenging, extend your arms as you lie on your front. Now lift your head, shoulders and arms as high as you can and lower with control.

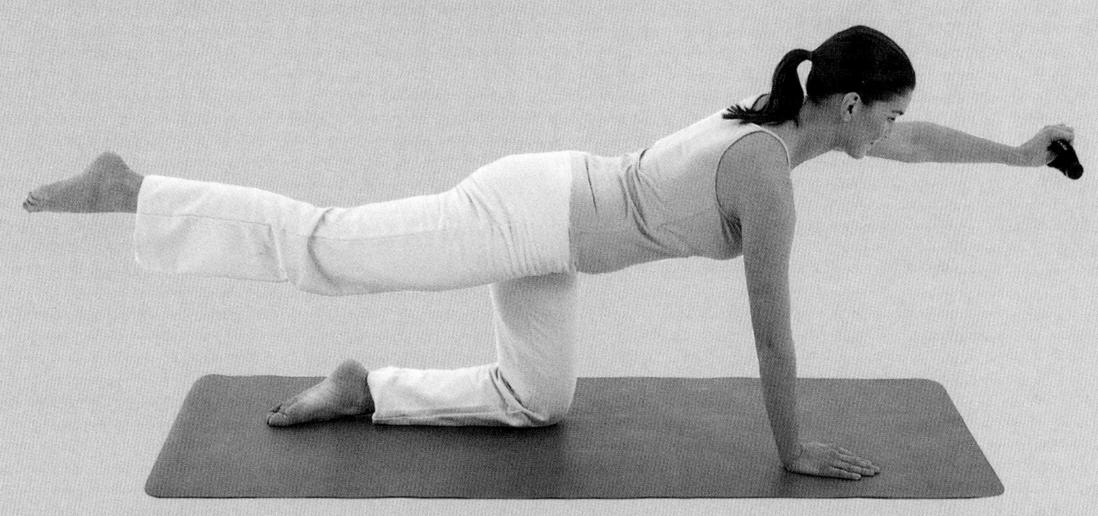

▲ All-fours superman 3

1 Again, perform the All-Fours Superman 1 balance exercise on page 52 but this time grasp a weight in one hand then lift this arm and opposite leg off the floor as before. Your shoulder muscle will be working hard to lift the weight, while your torso muscles will be working to maintain your balance.

2 Do 2 lifts on each side, holding each lift for 5 seconds.

▼ All-fours superman 2

1 Perform the All-Fours Superman 1 balance exercise on page 52 but this time, if you can, get someone to place a stick along the length of your back. Now as you slowly lift one arm and the opposite leg off the floor, keep your abdominal and back muscles tight to ensure they stay absolutely still so the stick does not roll off.

2 Repeat the exercise, lifting the other leg and arm.

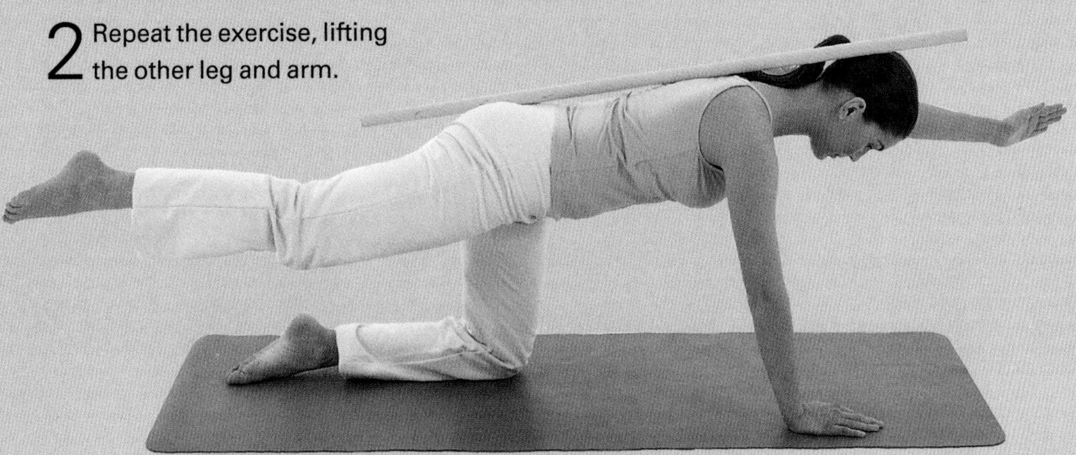

INCREASED FLEXIBILITY

You will have encountered various stretches throughout the programmes in this book, many of which are held for 8–10 seconds to allow the muscles to return to their pre-exercise length (see page 18). There are other types of stretching, however, which, rather than just return the muscles to their original length, actually aim to extend them and the boundaries of your flexibility. These include developmental stretching, stretching with a partner and PNF (proprioceptive neuro-muscular facilitation) stretching.

Developmental stretching

One of the best ways to extend your stretch routine is developmental stretching. This means exactly what it says – developing the stretch from the starting point to a further point. In order to hold the further position, you usually have to tense the opposing muscles to keep you there. This struggle creates a lot of body heat and is hard work.

Try some developmental stretches and see what a difference they make to your flexibility. Don't forget, that in order to do effective and safe stretching you must be warm (see page 19), and always make sure that the position you are in as you develop your stretch is supported. You should avoid any possibility of slipping out of position as this could cause injury.

Following the technique in the example shown here, take the developmental approach with any of the stretches from the stretch sections in this book, particularly Sit and Lean (see page 74), Lie and Lean (see page 75), First Stretch and Second Stretch (see page 92).

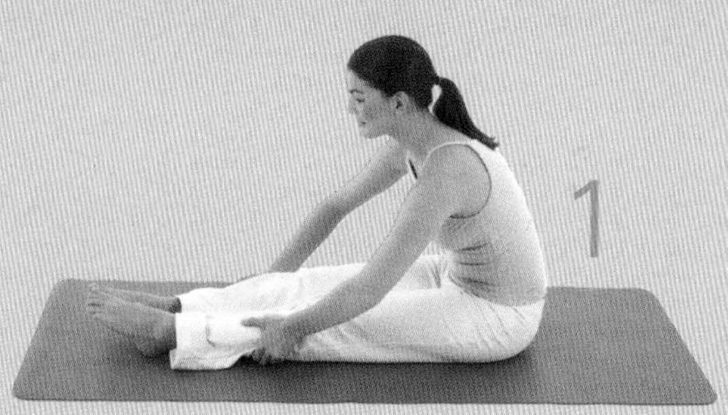

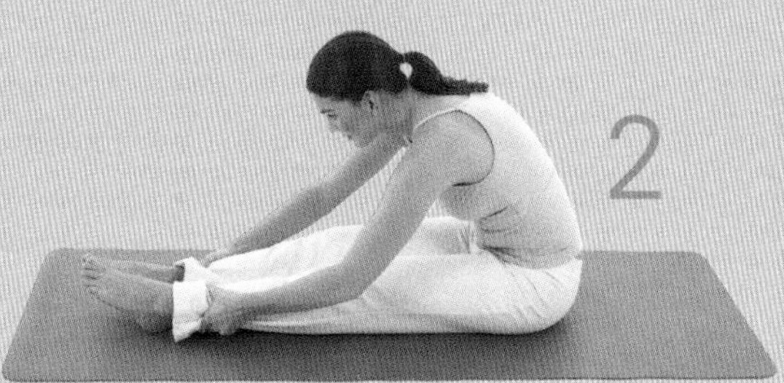

Developmental stretch

1 Sit on the floor with your legs outstretched. Sit up straight, lifting up and out of the ribcage, now start to inch your hands forward. Reach as far forward as you can until your body tells you to stop.

2 At this point you are attempting to extend the limit of your stretch still further so instead of withdrawing from the stretch as you normally would, stay in this position a little longer than feels comfortable. As the discomfort begins to recede – usually after about 20–30 seconds – your muscles should begin to 'give' a little, and you can try to take the position further by carefully leaning forward a little further. This resulting position is further than you thought you could go! Eventually, with practice, you may be able to stay in the stretch position for 1–2 minutes.

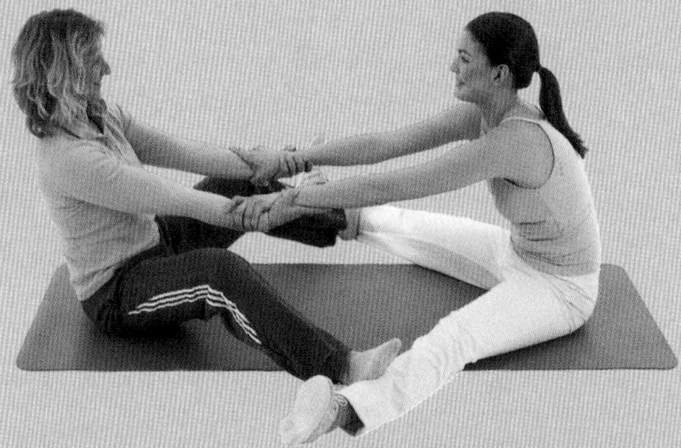

2 Partner stretching

Stretching with a partner is an enjoyable way to pursue your stretch goals. You can work with anyone who is a similar size to you, even if your flexibility levels are different. You must make sure that you are both concentrating and working seriously to help each other. The idea of having a partner is to allow that person to extend your stretch – gently – for you. He/she will use their strength to support you so that you are safely guided into a deeper stretch. Extra body weight applied can aid the stretcher into a more comfortable position and with sustained pressure, help the muscles stretch further. You must, however, communicate well between you so that everything is clearly understood and certain limits are not exceeded.

PNF stretching

This type of stretching means extending the stretch by 'fooling' the muscles into relaxing a little more. This is possible because when you work a muscle against force for 30–50 seconds, its tone briefly drops immediately afterwards. When a stretch is then applied you will be able to take it a little further than you thought possible. This type of stretching must be done carefully and with adequate support for the body. Try the example shown.

3 PNF stretch

1 Lie on your back and lift one leg up toward your face, as far toward you as it will go. Take hold of this leg with both hands and note where your limit is. Now, using the force of your front thigh muscle, try to force the leg down towards the floor, but at the same time resist this force with your hands and keep the leg where it is.

2 Maintain this struggle of wills (and muscles) for up to 50 seconds, then release the tension. At this point pull the leg further in toward your body. You should find the leg will come much more easily toward you than it did before.

1

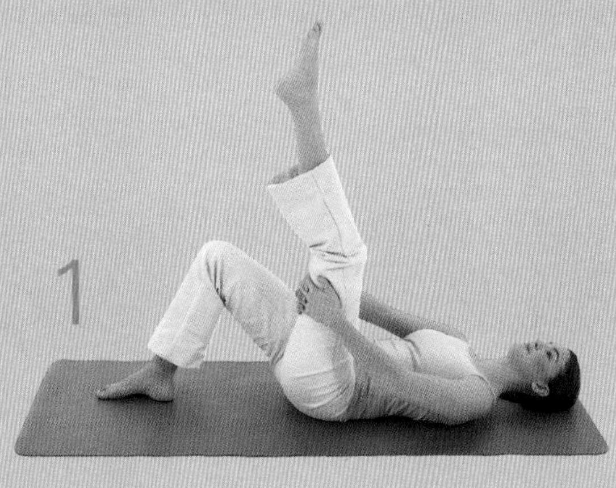

2

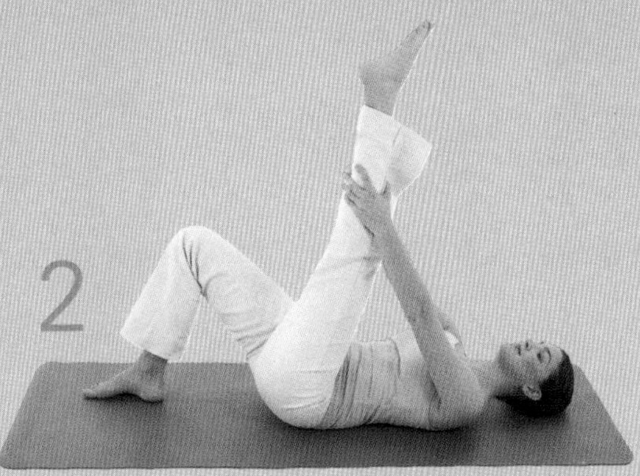

INDEX

acknowledgements

Executive editor Doreen Pallamartschuk-Gillon
Project editor Alice Tyler

Executive art editor Rozelle Bentheim
Designer Peter Gerrish
Illustrations Bounford.com

Photographer Peter Pugh-Cook
Models Ceri Evans and Kaaren Buchanan

Senior production controller Jo Sim